Schering Foundation Workshop 6

Transgenic Animals as Model Systems for Human Diseases

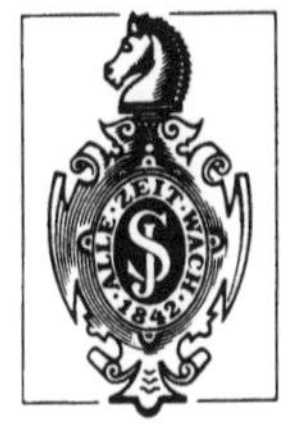

Schering Foundation Workshop

Editors: Günter Stock
Ursula-F. Habenicht

Vol. 1
Bioscience ⇌ Society
Workshop Report
Editors: D. J. Roy, B. E. Wynne, R. W. Old

Vol. 2
Round Table Discussion on Bioscience ⇌ Society
Editor: J. J. Cherfas

Vol. 3
Excitatory Amino Acids and Second Messenger Systems
Editors: V. I. Teichberg, L. Turski

Vol. 4
Spermatogenesis – Fertilization – Contraception
Editors: E. Nieschlag, U.-F. Habenicht

Vol. 5
Sex Steroids and the Cardiovascular System
Editors: P. Ramwell, G. Rubanyi, E. Schillinger

Vol. 6
Transgenic Animals as Model Systems for Human Diseases
Editors: E. F. Wagner, F. Theuring

Schering Foundation Workshop 6

Transgenic Animals as Model Systems for Human Diseases

E. F. Wagner, F. Theuring, Editors

With 39 Figures

Springer-Verlag Berlin Heidelberg GmbH

ISBN 978-3-662-02927-5   ISBN 978-3-662-02925-1 (eBook)
DOI 10.1007/978-3-662-02925-1

© Springer-Verlag Berlin Heidelberg 1993
Originally published by Springer-Verlag Berlin Heidelberg New York in 1993
Softcover reprint of the hardcover 1st edition 1993

The use of general descriptive names, registered names, trademarks, etc. in this publication does not imply, even in the absence of a specific statement, that such names are exempt from the relevant protective laws and regulations and therefore free for general use.

Product liability: The publishers cannot guarantee the accuracy of any information about dosage and application contained in this book. In every individual case the user must check such information by consulting the relevant literature.

Typesetting: Data conversion by Springer-Verlag

21/3130–5 4 3 2 1 0 – Printed on acid-free paper

Preface

In late 1980, the first paper describing the introduction of cloned DNA into fertilized mouse eggs by microinjection was published. During the next few months, several groups reported the generation of transgenic mice achieving stable integration and some expression of foreign DNA. This technique attracted considerable attention in the following years when it became clear that the newly introduced genes were incorporated into the germline of mice and that some of the foreign genes were found to be efficiently expressed.

The ability to introduce genes into the germline of mice (and other mammals) and the successful expression of the inserted gene within an organism provides new insights and opportunities for biomedical research. Transgenic technologies constitute an increasingly improtant tool to study the regulation and function of genes within the intact organism. They can be applied to a variety of different fields to analyze, for example, disease processes initiated and/or caused by the expression of certain gene products, to examine aspects of tumor development and techniques can be used to introduce human genes into the mouse/rat/rabbit background to study their function and to provide alternatives for the large-scale production of important but rare proteins, such as hormones in the milk of transgenic animals.

The different experimental strategies employing either gain-of-function or loss-of-function approaches in particular through the use of homologous recombination in embryonic stem cells allow the generation of specific animal models for human diseases. The detailed analysis of the underlying molecular mechanisms will provide now insights into the genetic origin of certain diseases and will lead to a

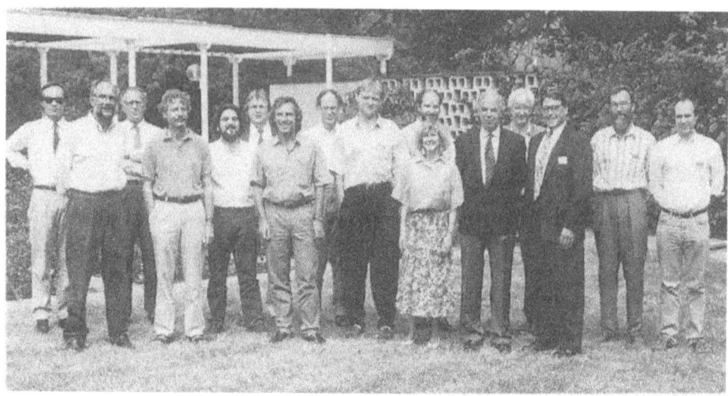

Abb. I. The participants of the workshop

better understanding of normal and abnormal physiological processes. This knowledge will improve also our diagnostic tools and will enhance the development of novel therapeutic interventions. We hope that this book will illustrate some of the current concepts used in transgenic research, emphasizing the application in the field of animal models for human diseases, and that it will serve as a basis to stimulate discussions for current and future basic and applied research.

Erwin F. Wagner
Franz Theuring

Contents

List of Contributors

Aguet, Michel
Institut für Molekularbiologie I, Universität Zürich, CH-8093 Zürich, Switzerland

Aguzzi, Adriano
Research Institute of Molecular Pathology (IMP), Dr. Bohr-Gasse 7, A-1030 Vienna, Austria

Arnold, Hans-Henning
Department of Toxicology, University of Hamburg Medical School, Grindelallee 117, W-2000 Hamburg 13, Germany

Büeler, Hansruedi
Institut für Molekularbiologie I, Universität Zürich, CH-8093 Zürich, Switzerland

Braun, Thomas
Department of Toxicology, University of Hamburg Medical School, Grindelallee 117, W-2000 Hamburg 13, Germany

Coffey, Robert J.
Department of Medicine, Vanderbilt University, Nashville, TN 37232, USA

Dempsey, Peter J.
Department of Medicine, Vanderbilt University, Nashville, TN 37232, USA

Fischer, Marek
Institut für Molekularbiologie I, Universität Zürich, CH-8093 Zürich, Switzerland

Furth, Priscilla A.
Department of Medicine, University of Maryland School of Medicine, Baltimore, MD 21201, USA

Ganten, Detlev
Max Delbrück Center for Molecular Medicine, W-1000 Berlin-Buch, Germany

Hennighausen, Lothar
Laboratory of Biochemistry and Metabolism, National Institutes of Health, Bethesda, MD 20892, USA

Hohmann, Christine F.
Molecular Neurogenetics Laboratory, 202 MRC, McLean Hospital, 115 Mill Street, Belmont, MA 02178, USA

Jaenisch, Rudolf
Whitehead Institute for Biomedical Research and Department of Biology, Massachusetts Institute of Technology, Nine Cambridge Center, Cambridge, MA 02142, USA

Kammerscheidt, Anja
Molecular Neurogenetics Laboratory, 202 MRC, McLean Hospital, 115 Mill Street, Belmont, MA 02178, USA

Kollias, George A.
Laboratory of Molecular Genetics, Hellenic Pasteur Institute, 127 Vas Sofias Av., Athens 115221, Greece

Kozlowski, Michael R.
Molecular Neurogenetics Laboratory, 202 MRC, McLean Hospital, 115 Mill Street, Belmont, MA 02178, USA

McKnight, Robert A.
Laboratory of Biochemistry and Metabolism, National Institutes of Health, Bethesda, MD 20892, USA

Neve, Rachael L.
Molecular Neurogenetics Laboratory, 202 MRC, McLean Hospital, 115 Mill Street, Belmont, MA 02178, USA

Paul, Martin
German Institute for High Blood Pressure Research, Department Pharmacology, University of Heidelberg, Im Neuenheimer Feld 366, W-6900 Heidelberg, Germany

Pursel, Vern G.
Mapping Laboratory, United States Department of Agriculture, Beltsville, MD 20705, USA

Rexroad, Caird Jr.
Mapping Laboratory, United States Department of Agriculture, Beltsville, MD 20705, USA

Rubin, Edward
Life Sciences Division, 1 Cyclotron Road, Lawrence Berkeley Laboratory, Berkeley, CA 94720, USA

Rudnicki, Michael A.
Whitehead Institute for Biomedical Research and Department of Biology, Massachusetts Institute of Technology, Nine Cambridge Center, Cambridge, MA 02142, USA

Schultz, Joshua
Life Sciences Division, 1 Cyclotron Road, Lawrence Berkeley Laboratory, Berkeley, CA 94720, USA

Shamay, Avi
Laboratory of Biochemistry and Metabolism, National Institutes of Health, Bethesda, MD 20892, USA

Wagner, Erwin F.
Research Institute of Molecular Pathology (IMP), Dr. Bohr-Gasse 7, A-1030 Vienna, Austria

Wagner, Jürgen
German Institute for High Blood Pressure Research, Department Pharmacology, University of Heidelberg, Im Neuenheimer Feld 366, W-6900 Heidelberg, Germany

Wall, Robert J.
Mapping Laboratory, United States Department of Agriculture, Beltsville, MD 20705, USA

Weissmann, Charles
Institut für Molekularbiologie I, Universität Zürich, CH-8093 Zürich, Switzerland

1 The Human Renin-Angiotensin System in Transgenic Rats – New Tools for Antihypertensive Therapy

Jürgen Wagner, Martin Paul, and Detlev Ganten

1.1 Introduction

The renin–angiotensin system (RAS) is one of the best studied regulatory systems involved in control of cardiovascular function and volume homeostasis. Its effector peptide angiotensin II exerts a multiplicity of functions by raising peripheral resistance through vasoconstriction, enhancing renal sodium reabsorption, facilitation of catecholamine release from sympathetic nerve endings or stimulation of mineralcorticoid production in the adrenal gland (Table 1) [1,2].

Table 1. Functions of angiotensin II in various tissues (adapted from [55])

Tissue	Function
Kidney	Renal blood flow, glomerlular filtration rate, sodium reabsorption
Vasculature	Vascular tone, hypertrophy
Heart	Contractility, hypertrophy
Adrenal gland	Aldosterone section, catecholamine release
Brain	Thirst, vasopressin and catecholamine release
Pituitary	ACTH, gonadotropin hormones, prolactin release
Ovary	Ovulation, estrogen production (?)
Uterus	Uteroplacental flow, contractility
Testes	Androgen production (?)
Gut	Ion and water absorption
Eye	Ocular blood flow (?)

These integrative functions focussing on control of body salt and water homeostasis as well as blood pressure have led to the hypothesis that malfunction of this system may be related to the pathogenesis of hypertension [3,4].

Since the 1940s it has been known that activation of the RAS may indeed raise blood pressure as in the case of two-kidney–one-clip hypertensive rats [5]. Unilateral renal ischemia leads to secretion of renin from the "clipped" kidney, resulting in enhanced angiotensin II formation and raised blood pressure. This model is known as a high-renin hypertensive model, which is similar to human hypertensives with renal artery stenosis. The subdivision of hypertensive patients according to their plasma renin levels in high-, normal- or low-renin hypertension groups underscores the relevance which has been attributed to this system in hypertension [6].

Due to the major role of the RAS in blood pressure control, it has been considered as a candidate gene system for hypertension. Recently, the angiotensin-converting-enzyme gene has been found in a region of the rat chromosome which is linked to the hypertensive phenotype in the stroke-prone strain of spontaneously hypertensive rats [7].

Studies on the tissue-specific regulation of gene expression of the components of the RAS in humans are difficult to perform due to ob-

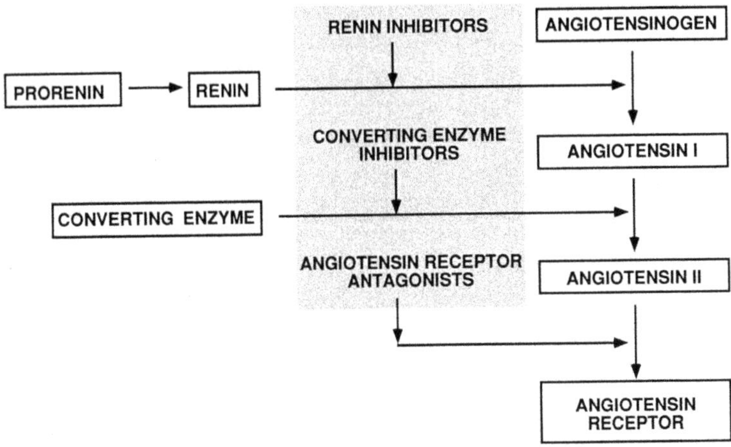

Fig. 1. Enzymatic cascade of the renin–angiotensin system (RAS). The reaction of renin with angiotensinogen to form angiotensin I is the rate-limiting step of the activation of the RAS. Renin inhibitors may block this highly species-specific reaction. The inactive decapeptid angiotensin I is cleaved to the effector peptide angiotensin II, which interacts with the angiotensin receptor. Both the formation of angiotensin II and its interaction with its receptor may be interrupted by non-species-specific converting-enzyme inhibitors or receptor antagonists, respectively

vious ethical reasons and the small amounts of tissue available, e.g., from biopsies [8,9]. Since all hypertension research is ultimately focussed on human hypertension and its treatment, the "transfer" of the human genes to the rat as a test model for cardiovascular research would be highly advantageous to investigate the role of the human RAS components in hypertension. Therefore, transgenic rats may be helpful to fully understand the regulation of the *human* genes of the RAS in vivo. It offers the possibility to study a hypertensive rat model, where blood pressure elevation is dependent on the interaction of the human RAS components and their enzyme kinetics.

That the RAS may not only be involved in the development of hypertension, but also influence the process of cardiac and vascular hypertrophy is suppported by a large body of data [10,11]. These primarily physiological adaptive responses to elevated blood pressure progress in the course of hypertension to cardiac and renal failure. Blood pressure-independent, mitogenic and growth-promoting effects of angiotensin II on endothelial cells, fibroblasts and vascular smooth muscle cells, possibly via activation of oncogenes, are well known [12–14]. These influences may mediate the deleterious maladaptations of the cardiovascular system.

Since coexpression of the components of the RAS has been demonstrated in the heart or the vasculature, angiotensin II formation in the cardiovascular system may not solely be derived from the plasma, but rather be produced by local, tissue-specific RAS and act on the surrounding tissue in a paracrine or autocrine fashion (see [15–17] for review). Expression of human renin and other components of the RAS in extrarenal tissues in transgenic rats may be a way to investigate the activity of tissue-specific human RAS on cardiovascular morphology and function.

Due to the widespread implications of the RAS in hypertension, an arsenal of pharmacological substances which interrupt this system on every step of the cascade has been developed (Fig. 1). The largest clinical experience has been obtained from angiotensin converting-enzyme inhibitors (CEI), which now belong to the most effective and safest antihypertensive drugs. Additionally, angiotensin receptor antagonists and renin inhibitors are now clinically being studied for their use in antihypertensive treatment [18–20].

Pharmacological studies using these substances, however, can not give a final answer as to the role of the RAS and also have clinical drawbacks: CEI, for example, are not specific for the RAS and cleave other vasoactive peptides, such as bradykinin. These may be responsible for some of the side effects of CEI such as painful cough [19]. Angiotensin receptor antagonists raise plasma angiotensin II concentration and may increase binding of angiotensin II to other angiotensin receptor subtypes not blocked by the particular antagonist and thus provoke unwanted side effects.

The rate-limiting step of the enzymatic cascade of the RAS is the reaction of human renin with its substrate angiotensinogen [21]. This highly specific reaction can be blocked by renin inhibitors. Potentially, blockade of this system at this early level could be therapeutically of advantage and may, at least theoretically, be superior to blockade of converting enzyme inhibiton generally or in selected cases [22]. However, the development of such renin inhibitors has been hampered by the species specificity of the renin substrate reaction. Angiotensinogen is cleaved between the aminoacids at position 10 and 11. At position 13 a histidine is substituted for a tyrosine in human angiotensinogen, which is probably responsible for the species specificity due to its charged group [23,24]. This precluded rats as test models, even though they are highly suitable for cardiovascular research and the testing of antihypertensive drugs. A large body of knowledge about the RAS could only be obtained by investigations performed in this animal species. Preclinical studies on renin inhibitors had to be restricted to primates such as marmosets or to humans in selected cases [20,25]. Transfer of the human renin substrate reaction to the rat would allow the usage of rats as test models for the development of human-specific renin inhibitors. Therefore transgenic rats carrying the human renin and angiotensinogen genes are tools to address these questions and to measure the endocrinological, hemodynamic and functional responses to human renin inhibitors acutely or after chronic administration, which may be of higher importance in hypertension research.

In the following, we report on the generation of transgenic rats harboring the human RAS components renin and angiotensinogen under their natural promoters and a human prorenin construct driven by a heterologous metallothionein promoter.

1.2 Generation of Transgenic Rats – Methodological Considerations

In transgenic experiments, foreign genes have been stably integrated into the genome of a number of species, such as mice, rats, goats, and swine, but mice have been used most extensively in transgenic research. Several factors may account for this: There is a large database of mouse genetics, and transgenic technology can easily be applied in this species. For some areas of research, however, the mouse may not be the most ideal species for transgenic studies. Its size puts limitations on the methodological arsenal which can be used for the detailed investigation of phenotypic changes induced by the expression of transgenes (Table 2). One area of research where this is particularly true is cardiovascular biology. Although investigators have succeeded in ap-

Table 2. Transgenic rats versus mice in cardiovascular research

Advantages of rats	
Large body of knowledge on rat physiology in hypertension	Physiology/pathophysiology Morphology Functional studies Long-term studies
Technical aspects	Acute/chronic instrumentation Telemetry Plethysmography (tail)
Parameters	Hemodynamic Endocrinological (hormone loevels, vasoactive peptides Organ function (cardiac, renal function)

Disadvantages of rats
Size
Costs
Comparatively low number of offspring
Long generation times
Microinjection procedure/hormonal treatment
Small data base of rat genetics

plying sophisticated techniques to the measurement of cardiovascular parameters in mice [26,27] this is still considered an exception.

In addition, primary hypertension, for example, is virtually unknown in mice, whereas a great number of rat strains show this disorder [28]. Experimental hypertension research, therefore, has largely been carried out using rats as a model and extensive data are available to serve as reference points for the measurement of cardiovascular parameters in this species. These considerations made it desirable to establish transgenic rats as experimental models in hypertension research. Transgenic animals are defined by the fact that new genetic material has been integrated in the genome by experimental methods other than breeding. Through incorporation into the germ cells, transgenic founder animals pass the transgene on to their offspring and a transgenic line can be established. There are a number of methods available to introduce genetic material into the genome of an animal. Retroviral infection of embryonic cells has been used to generate transgenic mice, but the most widely used method is microinjection of DNA into the pronucleus of a fertilized oocyte [29]. These cells are obtained from animals which have been mated after their ovulation had been stimulated by gonadotropin treatment. After microinjection, the oocytes are reimplanted into the oviduct or uterus of a pseudopregnant female, which had been mated with a vasectomized or sterile male. The offspring of this animal is then screened for the presence of the transgene, by extracting DNA from a small tissue sample, for example, a tail biopsy, and by its analysis using established methods such as Southern blotting and/or polymerase chain reaction [PCR) assays.

This general method can also be applied for the establishment of transgenic rats [30], but there are several technical details which have to be modified [31]. One is superovulation, which tends to be more difficult to achieve in the rat. This problem can be solved, however, by adapting the procedure of Armstrong and Opavsky [32] using the application of follicle-stimulating hormone (FSH) via osmotic minipump. By this approach the first transgenic rat line in cardiovascular research was established by Mullins, Peters, and Ganten [33], who expressed the mouse *Ren*-2 gene in rats.

1.3 Experimental Approaches to the Use of Transgenic Animals

Transgenic animals can be used to address different experimental questions. First, transgenic lines can be established with the purpose of adding an additional gene to develop models for the in vivo study of expression and regulation as well as possible phenotypic changes induced by the transgene. Another widely used application in transgenic research is the establishment of permanent cell lines derived from transgenic animals. For these experiments, a tissue-specific promoter is fused with a gene which has oncogenic potential. An example for such experiments is the work of Sigmund et al. [34,35], who linked the regulatory region of the mouse *Ren*-2 gene to the cDNA for the SV40 T antigen, which induces tumorigenesis, and generated transgenic mice expressing this chimeric construct. The animals showed tumor formation in kidney, adrenal gland, testis, and subcutaneous tissue [36]. The transformed cells, in addition to their ability to produce renin mRNA and to secrete renin protein, could be passaged without losing these features specific for juxtaglomerular cells. They may therefore provide adequate tissue culture models to study renin biosynthesis, processing and secretion.

A third application for transgenic animals is in the study of gene regulation in vivo. Typically, such a scenario calls for the establishment of transgenics expressing constructs which consist of the regulatory region of a gene under investigation linked to a reporter gene such as the luciferase gene. These constructs can be used for the transient transfection of cells in tissue culture as well as for the generation of transgenic animals. Studies can thus be carried out to investigate the tissue-specific responses to stimuli on the level of gene transcription, but also for many other questions such as the identification of cell- and tissue-specific regulatory mechanisms. Experiments investigating these mechanisms for the renin gene are described elsewhere in greater detail [37–40].

A fourth application of transgenic techniques is the establishment of whole animal models overexpressing a specific gene in the organism. To achieve this, a heterologous promoter inducing high levels of expression is linked to the gene or cDNA in question. Since extreme overexpression of genes in many cases will prove lethal during fetal life, inducible promoter sequences have proven to be more useful. These sequences show only little activity in the noninduced state, which allows it to prevent possible deleterious effects of transgene expression during ontogeny. Expression can be induced at a timepoint when the experimental protocol calls for the overexpression. One of the promoters used for such types of experiments is the metallothionein promoter, which can be induced by heavy metals such as zinc sulfate in the drinking water. This promoter has been used successfully to overexpress rat renin and angiotensinogen genes in transgenic mice [41].

1.4 Transgenic Rats Carrying Genes of the Human RAS

1.4.1 Transgenic Rats Harboring the Human Renin Gene

A construct containing the entire human renin gene was microinjected into the pronuclei of fertilized rat oocytes from outbred Sprague-Dawley. The construct comprised a total length of 17.6 kb after stripping it from vector-encoded sequences [42]. It contained 10 exons, 9 introns and 3 kb of 5'-flanking sequence and 1.2 kb of 3'-flanking sequence (Fig. 2). Two rat lines could be obtained which transmitted the transgene to their progeny [43].

These transgenic rats produced and secreted active human renin into their plasma, as has been determined by an immunoradiometric assay using monoclonal antibodies specific for human renin. The plasma levels of active human renin in one line was slightly less than in humans, whereas active human renin exceeded about twelve times the levels found in humans (1.5 ng ANGI/ml per hour; [44]) in the other.

To examine whether the presence of the transgene would interfere with the production of the endogenous host renin, plasma rat renin

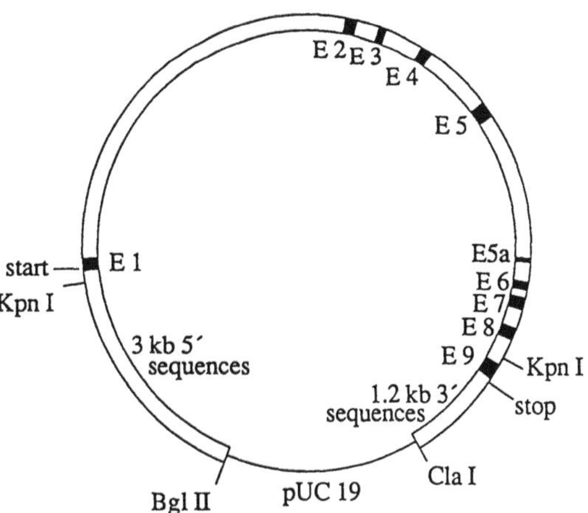

Fig. 2. Human renin gene construct. The genomic construct contained 3 kb of 5'-flanking and 1.2 kb of 3'-flanking region, ten exons and nine introns, having been stripped of vector sequences prior to microinjection [42,43]

concentration was also determined, but no significant differences existed between transgenic rats and negative controls. Also, no alterations in other components of the RAS such as angiotensin I, II or angiotensinogen could be detected. Consequently, both rats strains were normotensive at about 133 ± 3 mmHg as determined by tail plethysmography. These negative findings can be explained by the fact that human renin does not interact with rat angiotensinogen except at very high doses. To investigate how the human renin transgene responds to physiological stimuli of renin secretion, animals were sodium depleted by initial intraperitoneal injection of furosemide (10 mg/kg) and placement on a low-sodium diet for 3 days. In plasma, active human renin levels increased by about 11-fold up to $58.3 \pm 9x$ pg/ml, and rat renin slightly less by about eight times. This indicates, that the transgene is regulated by sodium depletion and does not interfere with rat renin production even under stimulated conditions.

Transgene expression was found to be highest in the kidney, but was also present in extrarenal tissues such as the lung or the gastrointestinal tract [43]. On the cellular level, in situ hybridization showed that human renin expression under basal conditions is confined to the juxtaglomerular apparatus.

These findings are comparable to data obtained from the mouse, in which human renin had also been expressed [42,45]. Transgene expression in the mouse was confined to the vas afferens of the kidney, with expression of renin approximately 7-fold higher than in humans, but still about ten times less than mouse renin.

1.4.2 Transgenic Rats Harboring Human Prorenin Under Control of the Metallothionein Promoter

Transgenic rats were generated using a minigene construct consisting of the metallothionein promoter, the complete human renin cDNA and intron, as well as polyA$^+$ sequences derived from the SV40 virus DNA. The purpose of this experiment was to study the effects of enhanced human renin expression in the rat under control of an inducible promoter. One of the questions to be answered by this experiment was to study the pathophysiological effects of increased plasma levels of human prorenin and active renin. Prorenin has been considered to play

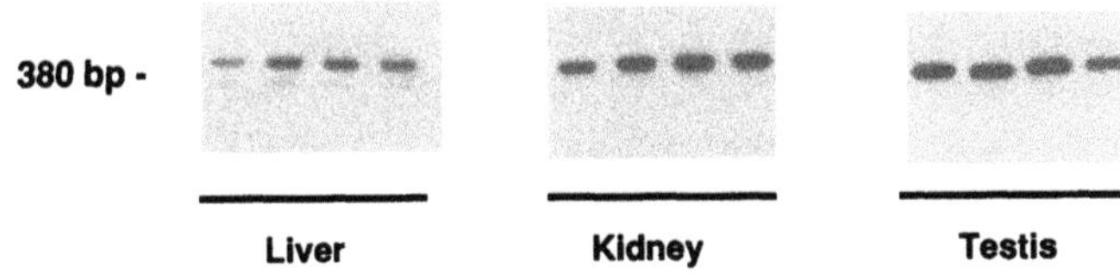

Fig. 3. Expression of human renin mRNA in tissues of transgenic rats carrying human renin under control of the metallothionein promoter. Human renin mRNA can be detected by a reverse transcription polymerase chain reaction (PCR) assay using human renin specific primers [9]. High expression of human renin mRNA in kidney, testis, and liver is indicated. Rat kidney total RNA from transgenic negative animals did not show a PCR signal (not shown). Total RNA was isolated after 2 weeks treatment with 25 mM ZnSO$_4$ in the drinking water

an important role for the overall function of the RAS [46]. It has been hypothesized that plasma prorenin may serve as a pool of the inactive enzyme which is circulating in the plasma and taken up to be activated at the tissue site. Other reports have postulated that prorenin may have additional functions in several organs, for example, the genital tract [47,48]. This led to the hypothesis that overexpression of prorenin alone could have pathophysiological consequences. After obtaining founder animals using the above mentioned construct, the transgenic rats were bred until an F3 generation was obtained. After screening for the presence of the transgene, eight heterozygous animals (5 female, 3 male) were subjected to further studies. Animals were screened for human prorenin and active renin concentrations in plasma following enhancement of gene expression by heavy metal feeding (14 days on 25 mM ZnSO$_4$ in the drinking water). After treatment, prorenin concentrations in the plasma were 110 pg/ml $\pm$ 6.6 SEM ($n=8$), whereas only small concentrations of active human renin (ranging from 2 to 7 pg/ml) could be detected. The transgene was expressed in a number of tissues. A species-specific PCR showed human renin mRNA to be present in many organs, with particularly high concentrations in liver, kidney, and testis (Fig. 3). A quantitative assay for human renin [9] was then applied to quantify the human renin mRNA concentrations in these organs (Fig. 4). Highest concentrations were found in the testis (1.7 pg renin/μg total RNA), followed by the kidney (0.21 pg renin/μg

LIVER

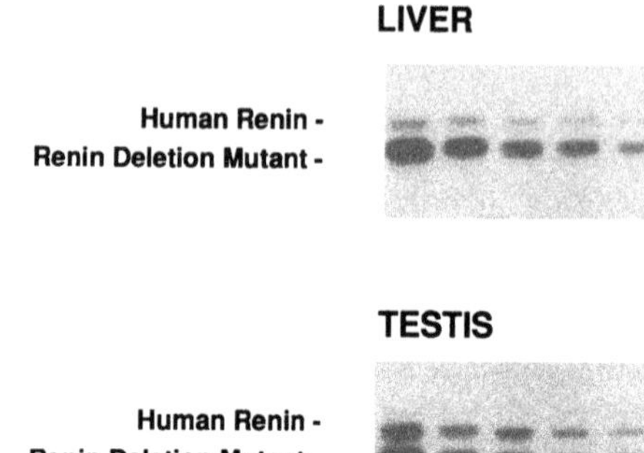

Fig. 4. Quantitative PCR assay for liver and testis of transgenic rats carrying the human renin gene under control of the metallothionein promoter. For quantification, a deletion mutant of the human renin gene, using the same primer binding sites as the human renin transgene, is coamplified as an internal standard. After gel electrophoresis, transgenic human renin and deletion mutant cDNA amplification products can be separated by size. A dilution curve of the PCR samples is used for regression analysis [9]. At the same amount of mutant molecules used, the higher signal intensity of the human renin transgene PCR product in testis as compared to liver indicates a higher expression of the human renin transgene in testis (1.7 pg renin/µg total RNA) than in liver (0.035 pg renin/µg total RNA)

total RNA) and liver (0.035 pg renin/µg total RNA). Analysis of cardiovascular parameters such as arterial blood pressure in these animals did not reveal any significant alterations compared to nontransgenic controls.

The concentrations of human prorenin in the plasma of these transgenic animals was found to be low compared to humans or rats, indicating that the construct used for the generation of these animals did not provide an actual overexpression of prorenin or active renin. Therefore, the highly interesting question of whether prorenin alone – independent of active renin – has physiological effects remains open. However, important lessions can be learned from these experiments: Stronger promoters such as viral LTR sequences may be needed to achieve higher levels of secretion of human prorenin into the plasma of transgenic rats. Additionally, if correct renin biosynthesis is the goal, promoters should also be chosen which direct expression into cells that have the appropriate intracellular apparatus to correctly process and secrete prorenin and active renin.

1.4.3 Transgenic Rats Harboring the Human Angiotensinogen Gene

The genomic human angiotensinogen gene construct, comprising five exons, four introns, 1.3 kb of 5'-flanking region and 2.4 kb of 3'-flanking region, was used to generate transgenic rats carrying the human angiotensinogen transgene (Fig. 5) [49]. Four lines could be obtained which transmitted the transgene to their progeny. Human angiotensinogen was secreted into the plasma in all rats but the levels markedly varied between the lines ranging from 120 g/ml up to 5 mg/ml. Thus, all four lines exceeded plasma angiotensinogen levels in humans which amounts to about 60 μg/ml [50].

Despite the high plasma levels, these animals were normotensive, indicating that human angiotensinogen did not interact with rat renin.

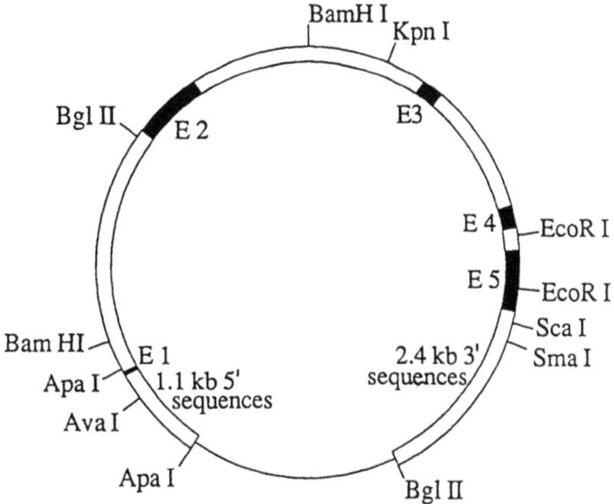

Fig. 5. Human angiotensinogen gene construct. The entire human angiotensinogen gene containing 1.1 kb of 5'-flanking sequences, five exons, four introns, and 2.4 kb of 3'-flanking region were microinjected without vector sequences [49]

Compared to transgene negative controls, rat angiotensinogen and angiotensin II levels were not significantly different in transgenics.

Transgene expression was highest at the appropriate sites in the liver, where it was expressed in the parenchyma. Transgene expression was also detected about tenfold lower in the kidney or the gastrointestinal tract. These findings are in contrast to a previously described transgenic mouse strain carrying the human angiotensinogen gene. Here, human angiotensinogen was expressed as high in the kidney as in the liver, in contrast to humans, in whom kidney angiotensinogen expression is low [51]. The reasons for these differences in the quantity of tissue-specific expression are not completely understood, but it may be due to the lack of negatively regulatory sequences beyond the 1.3 kb of 5'-flanking region, which might be necessary to suppress renal angiotensinogen expression.

1.5 Extrarenal Expression of Human Transgenes

Classically, the RAS has been viewed at as an endocrine system where the active components are produced in the kidney (renin), liver (angiotensinogen), and lung (converting enzyme) (Fig. 1). These are then secreted into the plasma, where they produce blood-borne angiotensin II that finally exerts its effects on the target organs (Table 1). However, the blood pressure-lowering effect of captopril in low-renin hypertension or in dialysis patients, who have lost the ability to produce active renin from the kidneys, as well as the demonstration of plasma prorenin levels after nephrectomy, which are sometimes as high as in humans with normal kidneys, pointed towards an extrarenal production of renin [15,52].

Renin expression could be detected in a number of other tissues such as the brain, the adrenals, or the vasculature as well as in tissues which appear not to be primarily involved in cardiovascular regulation as in the gastrointestinal tract. Similarly, angiotensinogen and converting enzyme expression is widespread [53,54]. The coexistence of all the components of the RAS in one tissue has raised the hypothesis that angiotensin II can be produced locally independent from the circulatory RAS and acts in an autocrine or paracrine fashion in the surrounding tissue [55]. Such extrarenal, local RAS have been suggested for the

Table 3. Tissue-specific expression of human renin and human angiotensinogen in transgenic rats. Coexpression of both transgenes is found in the kidney, but also in extrarenal tissues such as the adrenal, the brain, the gastrointestinal tract, or the lung. mRNA determinations have been performed by RNase protection assays using specific probes for human renin and angiotensinogen, respectively [43]

Human	Renin	Angiotensinogen
Kidney	+	+
Liver	−	+
Heart	−	+
Adrenal	+	+
Lung	+	+
Jejunum	+	+
Spleen	+	−
Brain	+[a]	+

[a] By RNase protection only detectable in line TGR(hREN)1988, by PCR also in line TGR(hREN)1936.

brain, the adrenal, the cardiovascular, and genitourinary system [15]. The transgenic rats, carrying the mouse *Ren-2* gene (see elsewhere in this book), exhibit high blood pressure in the presence of low plasma but enhanced tissue-specific RAS activity. This strengthens the contribution of the local RAS to the development of hypertension.

Human renin and angiotensinogen in transgenic rats have been shown to be expressed highest in the kidney or the liver. But expression is also demonstrable in extrarenal or extrahepatic tissues, respectively. Thus, human renin-mRNA is also present in the adrenals, the brain, the gastrointestinal tract, or the thyroid as well as in the lung (Table 3). In humans, renin expression in the gastrointestinal tract could be detected [56]. Angiotensinogen can be found extrahepatically in the lung, the gastrointestinum, brain areas and the heart (Table 3). The coexpression of the human transgenes in these organs supports the possibility of local angiotensin I production due to the interaction of the human proteins. Finally, angiotensin II can then be synthesized in presence of (non-species-specific) converting enzyme. The functional role of such human-dependent tissue-specific RAS remains to be established, but raises the question about the participation of tissue-specific RAS in human hypertension.

1.6 Species Specificity of the Human Renin Substrate Reaction – Effect of the Human Renin Inhibitor Ro 42-5892

Despite the high expression of the human transgenes, the rats remained normotensive as an indication of the species specificity of the human renin substrate reaction. As demonstrated by the unaltered levels of angiotensin II in both human renin and angiotensinogen transgenic rats, neither rat renin reacted with human angiotensinogen nor did human renin and rat angiotensinogen. Blood pressure remained unaltered, when the human specific renin inhibitor Ro 42-5892 was given as a bolus injection at a dosage of 1.5 mg/kg body weight to sodium-depleted TGR(hREN)1936 rats, whereas the angiotensin II receptor antagonist lowered blood pressure by about 20 mmHg. In contrast, $10^{-6}\,M$ Ro 42-5892 completely inhibited active human renin after incubation of plasma from sodium-depleted human renin transgenic rats, whereas rat renin remained unaffected. These findings show that human renin transgene does not add to blood pressure maintenance even after stimulation.

The species specificity of the human renin substrate reaction in the transgenic rats could further be demonstrated by injection of recombinant human renin into rats carrying the human angiotensinogen gene. Here, at a dosage of 5 µg ANG l/ml per hour, blood pressure rapidly increased from 142 ± 4 mmHg to 192 ± 8 mmHg. Addition of the human renin inhibitor Ro 42-5892 rapidly normalized the blood pressure to pretreatment values. Human renin at this dosage did not elicit a hypertensive response in transgene negative controls, indicating that the blood pressure increase was due to the interaction of human renin with human angiotensinogen (Fig. 6).

Infusion of *rat* renin in equipressor doses raised blood pressure as well, but in this case, Ro 42-5892 remained without any effect, whereas DuP 753 (10 mg/kg) normalized blood pressure rapidly, providing evidence that angiotensin II formation in this case originated from the reaction of rat renin with rat angiotensinogen (Fig. 6).

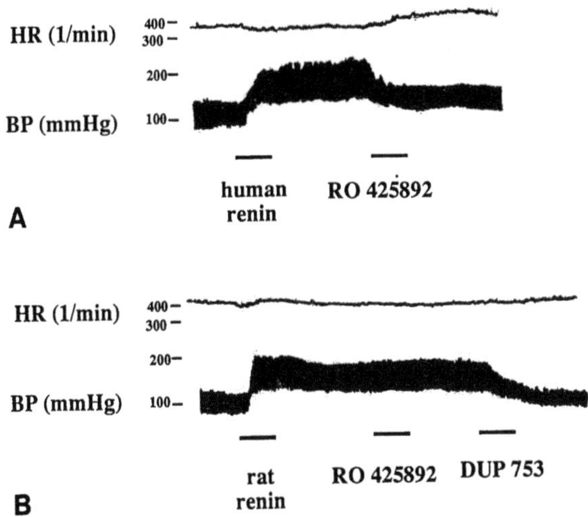

Fig. 6A,B. Specificity of the human renin substrate reaction. **A** Human renin infusion into transgenic rats carrying the human angiotensinogen gene elicits a hypertensive response which can rapidly be normalized by 1.5 mg/kg of the human renin-specific renin inhibitor Ro 42-5892. **B** Infusion of rat renin in equipressor doses also elevated blood pressure, but here, Ro 42-5892 remained without effect, whereas DuP 753 rapidly lowered blood pressure to pretreatment values. This indicates that the blood pressure increase in response to human renin is due to the interaction of human renin with human angiotensinogen, which can specifically be blocked by the human renin inhibitor in vivo [43]. *HR*, heart rate; *BP*, blood pressure

Pretreatment of TGR(hAOGEN) with Ro 42-5892 completely blocked the hypertensive response as well as the increase in angiotensin II formation after injection of human renin (see Fig. 7A,B). Ro 42-5892 alone neither lowered blood pressure below controls nor did it alter angiotensin II levels. The presence of DuP 753 (10 mg/kg i.v.) also prevented a blood pressure peak in presence of human renin.

The maintenance of the human-specific renin substrate reaction after chronic expression of the human renin or angiotensinogen transgenes allows the testing of renin inhibitors and their enzyme kinetics both in vitro and in vivo.

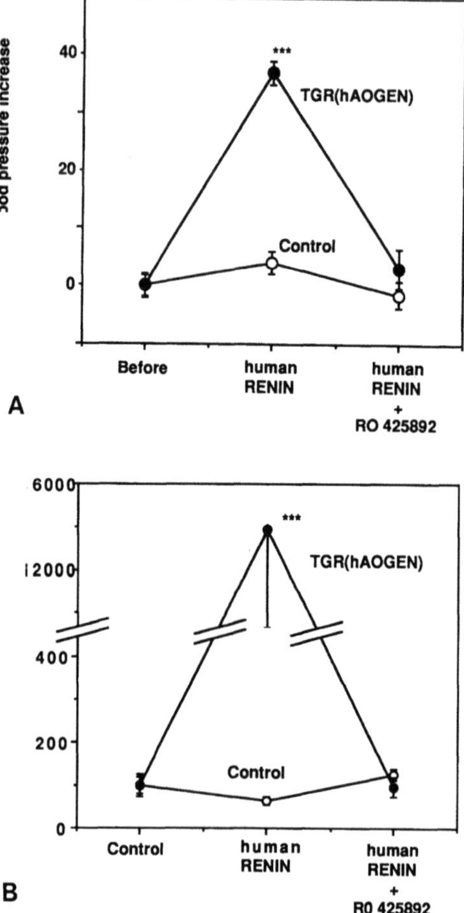

Fig. 7A,B. In vivo specificity of the human renin– angiotensinogen interaction. Infusion of human renin into transgenic rats carrying the human angiotensinogen markedly raises blood pressure. Pretreatment of transgenic rats 3 h prior to human renin infusion completely blocked blood pressure response (**A**). Plasma angiotensin II levels parallel the increase in blood pressure an are completely normal in presence of Ro 42-5892 (**B**). In transgenic negative controls, no increase in blood pressure or angiotensin II is observed after infusion of human renin at the applied dose

1.7 Conclusions

The general applicability of the transgenic rat model for basic research in cardiovascular biology and hypertension has now been established. This model offers advantages over the use of transgenic mice, particularly with respect to the characterization of cardiovascular parameters and pharmacological interventions, which are more readily available in this model. One of the first candidate systems thought to be involved in the pathogenesis of hypertension has been the RAS. The generation of rats expressing the human genes for renin and angiotensinogen have provided important models not only for the study of regulatory mechanisms of these genes, but also for the detailed investigation of possible pathophysiological effects of its expression. Ultimately, the information obtained from the study of these transgenic animals should provide important insights into the regulation of the RAS in man. In addition, they are also experimental systems to study the pharmacological effects of specific substances interfering with the RAS in humans, such as renin inhibitors. Such experiments have the potential of providing important information for the clinical use of these drugs, especially if they also influence specific sequelae of hypertension such as cardiac or vascular hypertrophy. Furthermore, the information that will be derived from future studies of those animals can be used to design experiments, which will further enhance our understanding of tissue-specific gene expression and regulation using chimeric constructs composed of the human renin and angiotensinogen promoters and reporter genes. Experiments will also focus on the investigation of other candidate genes thought to be involved in human hypertension, such as the genes for angiotensin-converting enzyme and for the ANG II receptor.

Acknowledgments. We gratefully acknowledge the supply of transgenic rats carrying the human renin gene under control of the metallothionein promoter from Dr. R. Movva, Dr. K. Bürki, Dr. N. Cook, and Dr. M. L. Park from the Department of Preclinical Research, Sandoz AG, Basel, Switzerland.

References

1. Vecsei P, Hackenthal E, Ganten D (1978) The renin-angiotensin-aldosterone system. Past, present and future. Klin Wochenschr 56 (Suppl I):5–21
2. Klett C, Hellmann W, Hackenthal E, Ganten D (1990) Pathophysiologie des Renin-Angiotensin-Systems. Wiener Med Wschr 140:2–11
3. Bader M, Kreutz R, Wagner J, Zeh K, Böhm M, Paul M, Ganten D (1992) Primary hypertension and the renin angiotensin system: from the laboratory experiment to clinical relevance. In: Colloque INSERM, vol 218: Genetic Hypertension. John Libbey Eurotext, Montrouge, London 359–370
4. Williams GH (1988) N Engl J Med 323:1517–1525
5. Goldblatt H, Lynch J, Hanzal RF, Summerville WW (1934) The production of persistent elevation of systolic blood pressure by means of renal ischemia. J Exp Med 59:347–379
6. Laragh JH, Sealey JE (1990) The renin-angiotensin-aldosterone system in hypertensive disorders: A key to two forms of arteriolar vasoconstriction and a possible clue to the risk of vascular injury (heart attack and stroke) and prognosis In: Laragh JH, Brenner BM (eds) Hypertension: pathophysiology, diagnosis and treatment. Raven, New York
7. Hilbert P, Lindpaintner K, Beckmann JS, Serikawa T , Soubrier F, Dubay C, Cartwright P, DeGouyon B, Julier C, Takahasi S, Vincent M, Ganten D, Georges M, Lathrop GM (1991) Chromosomal mapping of two genetic loci associated with blood-pressure regulation in hereditary hypertensive rats. Nature 353:521–529
8. Bruneval P, Fournier JG, Soubrier F, Belair MF, DaSilva JL, Guettier C, Pinet F, Tardivel I, Corvol P, Bariety J, Camilleri JP (1988) Detection and localization of renin messenger RNA in human pathologic tissues using in situ hybridization. Am J Pathol 131:320–330
9. Wagner J, Paul M, Ganten D, Ritz E (1991) Gene expression and quantification of components of the renin-angiotensin-system from human renal biopsies by the polymerase chain reaction. J Am Soc Nephrol 2:421 (Abstr)
10. Krieger JE, Dzau VJ (1991) Molecular biology of hypertension. Hypertension 18 (Suppl I):I–3–I–17
11. Morishita R, Higaki J, Miyazaki M, Ogihara T (1992) Possible role of the vascular renin-angiotensin system in hypertension and vascular hypertrophy. Hypertension 19 (suppl II):II–62–II–67
12. Schelling P, Fischer H, Ganten D (1991) Angiotensin and cell growth: a link to cardiovascular hypertrophy? J Hypertens 9:3–15
13. Paquet JL, Baudouin-Legros M, Brunelle G, Meyer (1990) Angiotensin II-induced proliferation of aortic myocytes in spontaneously hypertensive rats. J Hypertens 8:565–572
14. Taubman MB, Berk BC, Izumo S, Tsuda T, Alexander RW, Nadal-Ginard B (1989) Angiotensin induces c-fos mRNA in aortic smooth muscle:Role

of Ca2+ mobilization and protein kinase C activation. J Biol Chem 264:526–530

15. Paul M, Bachmann J, Ganten D (1992) The tissue renin-angiotensin systems in cardiovascular disease. Trends Cardiovasc Med 2:94–99
16. Lindpaintner K, Jin M, Wilhelm MJ, Suzuki F, Linz W, Schoelkens BA, Lang RE, Unger T, Ganten D (1988) Intracardiac generation of angiotensin and its physiological role. Circulation 77:I-18-I-23
17. Baker KM, Booz GW, Dostal DE (1992) Cardiac actions of angiotensin II: role of an intracardiac renin-angiotensin system. Ann Rev Physiol 54:227–241
18. Rhaleb NE, Rouissi N, Nantel F, D'Orleans-Juste P, Regoli D (1991) DuP 753 is a specific antagonist for the angiotensin receptor. Hypertension 17:480–484
19. Poole MD, Postman DS (1991) Characterization of cough associated with converting enzyme inhibitors. Otolaryngol Head Neck Surgery 105:714–716
20. van den Meiracker AH, Admiraal PJJ, Man in't Veld AJ, Derkx FHM, Ritsema van Eck HJ, Mulder P, Van Brummelen P, Schalekamp MADH (1990) Prolonged blood pressure reduction by orally active renin inhibitor RO 42-5892 in essential hypertension. Br Med J 301:205–210
21. Sealey JE, Laragh JH (1990) In: Laragh JH, Brenner BM (eds) Hypertension: Pathophysiology, Diagnosis and Management. Raven, New York, pp 1287–1318
22. Corvol P, Chauveau D, Jeunemaitre X, Menard J (1990) Human renin inhibitor peptides. Hypertension 16:1–11
23. Evans DB, Cornette JC, Sawyer TK, Staples DJ, De Vaux AE, Sharma SK (1990) Substrate specificity and inhibitor structure activity relationships of recombinante human renin: implications in the in vivo evaluation of renin inhibitors. Biotechnol Appl Biochem 12:161–175
24. Tewksbury DA, Dart RA, Travis J (1981) The amino terminal amino acid sequence of human angiotensinogen. J Biochem Biophys Res Commun 99:1311–1315
25. Ii Y, Murakami E, Hiwada K (1991) Effect of renin inhibitor, ES-8891, on renal renin secretion and storage in the marmoset: comparison with captopril. J Hypertens 9:1119–1125
26. Mockrin SC, Dzau VJ, Gross KW, Horan MJ (1991) Transgenic animals: new approaches to hypertension research. Hypertension 17:394–399
27. Field LJ (1991) Cardiovascular research in transgenic animals. Trends Cardiovasc Med 1:141–146
28. Ganten D, Lindpaintner K, Ganten U, Peters J, Zimmermann F, Bader M, Mullins J (1991) Transgenic rats: New animal models in hypertension research. Hypertension 17:843–855
29. Palmiter RD, Brinster RL (1986) Germ-line transformation of mice. Ann Rev Genet 20:465–499

30. Wagner J, Zeh K, Paul M (1992) Transgenic rats in hypertension research. J Hypertens 10:601–605
31. Mullins JJ, Ganten D. (1990) Transgenic animals: new approaches to hypertension research. J Hypertens 8 (Suppl 7):S35–S37
32. Armstrong DT, Opavsky MA (1988) Superovulation of immature rats by continuous infusion of FSH. Biol Reprod 39:511–518
33. Mullins JJ, Peters J, Ganten D (1990) Fulminant hypertension in transgenic rats harbouring the mouse Ren-2 gene. Nature 344:541–544
34. Sigmund CD, Gross KW (1990) Differential expression of the murine and rat renin genes in peripheral subcutaneous tissue. Biochem Biophys Res Commun 173:218–223
35. Sigmund CD, Jones CA, Jacob HJ, Ingelfinger J, Kim U, Gamble D, Dzau VJ, Gross KW (1991) Pathophysiology of vascular smooth muscle in renin promoter-T–antigen transgenic mice. Am J Physiol 260:F249–F257
36. Sigmund CD, Okuyama K, Ingelfinger J, Jones CA, Mullins JJ, Kane C, Kim U, Wu C, Kenny L, Rustum Y, Dzau VJ, Gross KW (1990) Isolation and characterization of renin-expression cell lines from transgenic mice containing a renin-promoter viral oncogene fusion construct. J Biol Chem 265:19916–19922
37. Paul M, Nakamura N, Pratt RE, Burt DW, Dzau VJ (1992) Cell dependent posttranslational processing and secretion of recombinant mouse renin-2. Am J Physiol 262:E224–E229
38. Sigmund CD, Gross KW (1991) Structure, expression, and regulation of the murine renin genes. Hypertension 18:446–457
39. Paul M, Burt DW, Krieger JE, Nakamura N, Dzau VJ (1992) Tissue specificity of renin promoter activity and regulation in mice. Am J Physiol 262:E644–E650
40. Nakamura N., Burt DW, Paul M, Dzau VJ (1989) Negative control elements and cAMP responsive sequences in the tissue-specific expression of mouse renin genes. Proc Natl Acad Sci USA 86:56–59
41. Ohkubo H, Kawakami H, Kakehi Y, Takumi T, Arai H, Yokota Y, Iwai M, Tanabe Y, Masu M, Hata J, Iwao H, Okamoto H, Yokoyama M, Nomura T, Katsuki M, Nakanishi S (1990) Generation of transgenic mice with elevated blood pressure by introduction of the rat renin and angiotensinogen genes. Proc Natl Acad Sci USA 87:5153–5157
42. Fukamizu A, Seo MS, Hatae T, Yokoyama M, Nomura T, Katsuki M, Murakami K (1989) Tissue-specific expression of the human renin gene in transgenic mice. Biochem Biophys Res Commun 165:826–832
43. Ganten D, Wagner J, Zeh K, Bader M, Michel JB, Paul M, Zimmermann F, Ruf P, Hilgenfeldt U, Ganten U, Kaling M, Bachmann S, Fukamizu A, Mullins JJ, Murakami K (1992) Species specificity of renin kinetics in transgenic rats harboring the human renin and angiotensinogen genes. Proc Natl Acad Sci USA

44. Menard J, Guyenne TT, Corvol P, Pau B, Simon D, Roncucci R (1985) Direct immunometric assay of active renin in human plasma. J Hypertens 3 (Suppl 3):S275–S278
45. Fukamizu A, Hatae T, Kon Y, Sugimura M, Hasegawa T, Yokoyama M, Nomura T, Katsuki M, Murakami K (1991) Human renin in transgenic mouse kidney is localized to juxtaglomerular cells. Biochem J 278:601–603
46. Sealey JE, Rubattu SA (1989) Prorenin and renin as separate mediators of tissue and circulating systems. Am J Hypertens 2:358–366
47. Glorioso N, Atlas SA, Laragh JH, Jewelewicz R, Sealey JE (1986) Prorenin in high concentrations in human ovarian follicular fluid. Science 233:1422–1424
48. Kim SJ, Shinjo M, Fukamizu A, Miyazaki H, Usuki S, Murakami K (1987) Identification of renin and renin messenger RNA sequence in rat ovary and uterus. Biochem Biophys Res Commun 142:169–175
49. Fukamizu A, Takahashi S, Seo MS, Tada M, Tanimoto K, Uehara S, Murakami K (1990) Structure and expression of the human angiotensinogen gene. J Biol Chem 265:7576–7582
50. Gardes J, Bouhnik J, Clauser E, Corvol P, Ménard J (1982) Role of angiotensinogen in blood pressure homeostasis. Hypertension 4:185–189
51. Takahashi S, Fukamizu A, Hasegawa T, Yokoyama M, Nomura T, Katsuki M, Murakami K (1991) Expression of the human angiotensinogen gene in transgenic mice and transfected cells. Biochem Biophys Res Commun 180:1103–1109
52. Sealey JE, White RP, Laragh JH, Rubin AL (1977) Plasma prorenin and renin in anephric patients. Circ Res 41 (Suppl II):17–21
53. Unger T, Gohlke P, Paul M, Rettig R (1991) Tissue renin-angiotensin systems: fact or fiction? J Cardiovasc Pharmacol 18 (Suppl 2):S20–S25
54. Dzau VJ, Pratt RE (1986) Renin-angiotensin system: biology, physiology, and pharmacology. The Heart and Cardiovasc Syst 2:1631–1662
55. Dzau VJ (1987) Implications of local angiotensin production in cardiovascular physiology and pharmacology. Am J Cardiol 59:59A–65A
56. Seo MS, Fukamizu A, Saito T, Murakami K (1991) Identification of a previously unrecognized production site of human renin. Biochim Biophys Acta 1129:87–89

2 Probing the Genetics
of Atherosclerosis in Transgenic Mice

Edward Rubin and Joshua Schultz

2.1 Murine Lipoproteins and Atherosclerosis

The mouse has long been thought to be a poor model for studying human lipoprotein metabolism and atherosclerosis. One of the major problems in using the mouse for these studies is that mice have significantly less total plasma cholesterol than do humans and do not develop atherosclerosis when fed the standard mouse chow diet containing 4 % fat and 0.2 % cholesterol. In addition, the lipoprotein profile of the mouse differs from that of humans in that most plasma cholesterol is transported as high density lipoprotein (HDL) while in humans low density lipoprotein (LDL) is the predominant lipoprotein species (Table 1). A major advance in developing the mouse as a model system for studying lipoprotein metabolism and atherosclerosis was the development of high fat (15 %) and high cholesterol (1 %–3 %) diets that could be tolerated by these animals for extended periods of time (Roberts and Thompson 1976; Paigen et al. 1985). When placed on these high fat diets the gross lipoprotein profile of the mouse re-

Table 1. Human and murine cholesterol and lipoprotein concentrations (mg/dl)

	Total cholesterol	VLDL + LDL cholesterol	LDL cholesterol
Human	210	170	40
Mice (C57)			
Chow	66	4	44
High fat	192	161	31

Human values were derived from normolipidemic subjects on Western style diets. The murine low fat chow diet contains 4.5% fat while the high fat diet has 15% fat.

sembles that of humans (Table 1). In addition, when subjected to these diets for 3–6 months certain inbred strains consistently develop atherosclerotic lesions in their proximal aorta (Paigen et al. 1987a; Stewart-Phillips et al. 1988; Paigen et al. 1990; Stewart-Phillips et al. 1991).

2.2 Lipoproteins and Atherosclerosis

Lipoproteins are macromolecular structures which transport non-polar lipids through the aquaeous vascular space. An illustration of a lipoprotein particle is shown in Fig. 1. Lipoproteins consist of a hydrophobic inner core containing cholesterol ester and triglycerides in varying amounts and are stabilized by a surrounding outside layer of phospholipid. Polar phospholipid head groups form the surface of these particles and interact with the aqueous environment of the intravascular space. Apolipoproteins and some free cholesterol are associated at the surface of lipoprotein particles and extend into the core. Apolipoproteins are a family of proteins which associate with lipoprotein particles and are characterized by the presence of the amphipathic α-helix, a secondary structural motif containing opposing polar and nonpolar faces oriented along the long axis of the helix. These repeating helical structures are responsible for the lipid affinity of apolipoproteins. The smallest of the major lipoprotein classes are the HDLs. HDL is composed of 50 % lipid and 50 % protein. Associated with

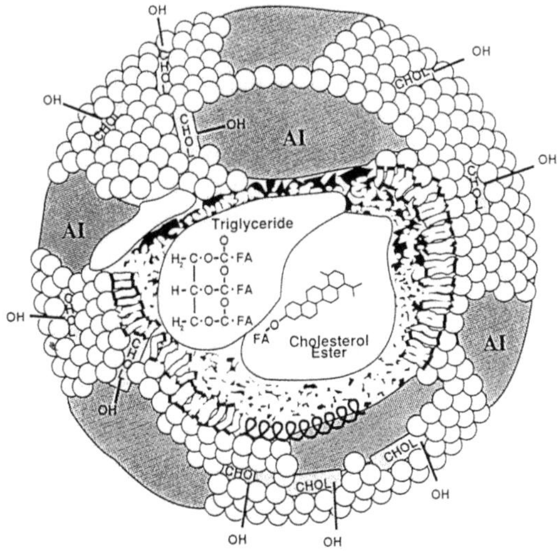

Fig. 1. Schematic diagram of a high-density lipoprotein (HDL). The core of these lipoprotein particles consist of triglyceride and cholesterol ester. Embedded in the surrounding outer layer of phospholipid (*white circles*) are molecules of cholesterol (CHOL–OH) and apolipoprotein AI (*shaded area*)

each HDL particle are several apolipoprotein molecules. The major HDL associated apolipoproteins include apolipoprotein apoAI (apoAI) and apolipoprotein AII (apoAII) which comprise 70 % and 20 % of HDL-associated apolipoproteins, respectively.

Plasma HDL concentrations as well as apoAI levels have been shown to be inversely correlated with the development of premature coronary heart disease (Glueck et al. 1976; Frager et al. 1979; Maciejko et al. 1983; Miller et al. 1987; Frohlich and Pritchard 1989). As its major apolipoprotein constituent, apoAI plays a central role in the synthesis and assembly of HDL particles. Deficiencies of apoAI result in low plasma HDL levels (Schaefer et al. 1982). In addition to its structural role, apoAI also serves as a cofactor for lecithin–cholesterol acyltransferase (LCAT), the enzyme responsible for cholesterol esterification in the plasma.

Discrete HDL size subclasses exist in human plasma (Gofman et al. 1950; Miller 1987; Nichols et al. 1989). Size differences between HDL subclasses are believed to result from the formation of thermodynamically stable HDL particles containing different apolipoprotein and lipid stoichiometries (Cheung et al. 1988). Human HDL particles also display apolipoprotein heterogeneity within specific subpopulations. Some particles contain apoAI with apoAII [Lp(AI w AII)] while others contain apoAI without apoAII [Lp(AI w/o AII)] (Cheung 1986). Separation of Lp(AI w AII) from Lp(AI w/o AII) by immunoaffinity chromatography has revealed size differences between these populations of particles (Cheung et al. 1988). HDL particles containing apoAII have a more constrained size distribution profile than particles which do not contain apoAII (Cheung and Albers 1984). The biological significance of HDL subpopulations remains unclear but may relate to interactions of specific HDL apolipoproteins with other components of lipid metabolism, including LCAT, cholesterol ester transfer protein (CETP), hepatic and lipoprotein lipases, and other plasma lipoproteins.

2.3 Apolipoprotein Studies with Human ApoAI Transgenic Mice

Since apoAI is believed to have a major effect on determining the level of HDL in plasma, the structure of the HDL particle, and on the susceptibility of an individual to develop atherosclerosis, we have examined the effect of altering the plasma levels of this protein in mice by producing animals transgenic for the human apoAI gene (referred to as AI transgenic mice). The human apoAI gene is located in a gene cluster containing apoCIII and apoAIV on chromosome 11 (Karathanasis 1985). The mouse apoAI cDNA has been cloned (Miller et al. 1983) and is located on mouse chromosome 9 (Lusis et al. 1983). Though the sequence of the mouse apoAI gene has not been reported, the rat and the human apoAI genes are similar in sequence and genomic organization, suggesting that the function of the rodent and human apoAI proteins have been conserved since the divergence of humans and primates (Haddad et al. 1986). The apoAII gene is located on chromosome 1 in both humans and mice (Lusis et al. 1983; Lackner et al. 1984). In humans and mice apoAI is synthesized in the liver and

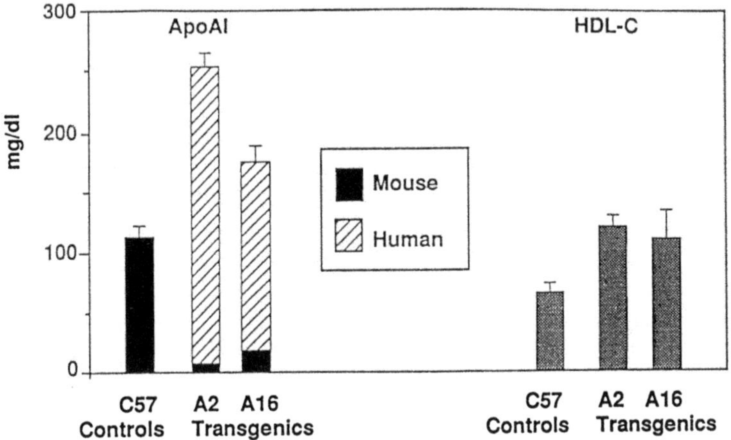

Fig. 2. ApoAI (*left*) and HDL cholesterol (*right*) concentrations in the plasma of C57BL/6 control and AI transgenic mice. Values shown represent the means and s.e.m. for 5–15 animals

small intestine whereas apoAII is found primarily in the liver (Eggerman et al. 1991).

In the following studies, we examined the effect of high apoAI expression by introducing the human apoAI gene into the atherosclerosis susceptible inbred mouse strain C57BL/6. An 11-kb human genomic fragment containing the entire human apoAI gene was used to construct several lines of AI transgenic mice. The human apoAI sequences were expressed exclusively in the livers of these animals. In the two independent human AI transgenic lines studied, plasma levels of total apoAI and HDL were increased to twice that of nontransgenic litter mates (Fig. 2). A surprising finding from these studies was that the level of endogenous apoAI in plasma from the transgenic animals is markedly reduced by up to tenfold and contributes only 4% to the total plasma apoAI mass. To investigate the mechanism for the decrease in plasma levels of mouse apoAI, total RNA was isolated from various tissues of transgenic and control animals and quantitation of murine apoAI mRNA levels was performed by northern blot analysis. Murine apoAI message was detected exclusively in the liver and the intestine of both groups of animals. Equal amounts of mouse apoAI mRNA

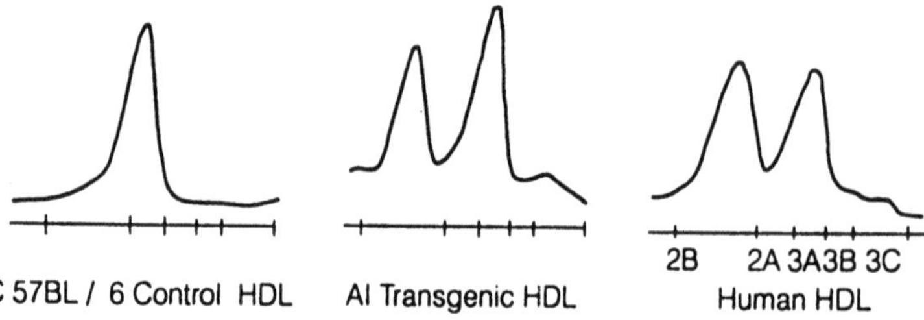

Fig. 3. Size distribution of HDL particles from C57BL/6 control, AI transgenic and human plasma. HDL particles were isolated from plasma and separtated by 4%–30% nondenaturing gradient gel electrophoresis. Shown are the computer-assisted densitometric scans of Coomassie Blue stained gels and the average mean particle diameters in nanometers

were quantitated in the tissues of transgenic and control animals, indicating that the marked decrease in murine plasma apoAI in the human AI transgenic mice is occurring at a posttranscriptional level. The model which we are presently entertaining and testing to explain the tenfold decrease in murine AI plasma levels is one that assumes that hybrid HDL particles containing both human and mouse apoAI are unstable. Subsequent degradation of the unstable hybrid particles leaves only stable human apoAI-containing particles, thereby decreasing the smaller pool of the endogenous apoAI.

Regardless of the mechanism responsible for the decreased plasma concentrations of the endogenous apoAI in human AI transgenic mice, these animals with human apoAI levels comprising greater than 95 % of the total plasma apoAI pool serve as a unique substrate in which to investigate the role that apoAI sequence plays in determining HDL size. In contrast to the single-sized HDL population present in control mice, human apoAI transgenic mice exhibit two distinct HDL populations identical in size to the human size subclasses HDL$_{2b}$ and HDL$_{3a}$ (Fig. 3). The size distribution of HDL particles composed almost entirely of human apoAI in the transgenic animals is indistinguishable from the size distribution of HDL isolated from the plasma of humans containing apoAI without apoAII. These results demonstrate the dominant role of the human apoAI sequence in determining the size of HDL particles regardless of whether the lipoprotein particles are formed in the plasma of humans or mice (Rubin et al. 1991).

We next turned our attention to examining the effect that changes in apoAI and HDL had on susceptibility to diet-induced atherosclerosis in these transgenic mice. In mice, atherosclerosis susceptibility is a polygenic trait involving the interaction of multiple genes. Athough no atherosclerosis susceptibility genes have been mapped to the murine apoAI gene, three genes (Ath-1, Ath-2, and Ath-3) have been identified in the mouse which do confer susceptibility to diet-induced atherosclerosis (Paigen et al. 1987b; Paigen 1989; Stewart-Phillips 1990; LeBoeuf et al. 1990). The C57BL/6 mice used for these studies are homozygous for atherosclerosis susceptibility alleles at all three of these loci and are therefore sensitive to diet-induced atherosclerosis. When fed a high fat diet the C57BL/6 strain differs from other strains resistant to diet-induced atherosclerosis by having lower HDL concentrations (Paigen et al. 1987a). Since numerous studies have demonstrated an association between low HDL concentrations and increased atherosclerosis susceptibility in humans, the lower HDL levels of C57BL/6 mice when placed on high fat diets are postulated to be responsible for their increased susceptibility to atherosclerosis. Therefore, the analysis of diet-induced atherosclerosis in the transgenic apoAI C57BL/6 animals with high apoAI and high HDL concentrations provides an approach to test the hypothesis that apoAI and HDL have direct antiatherogenic properties.

To quantitatively assess the effect of this genetic manipulation of apoAI levels on atherosclerosis we haved adapted the assay developed by Paigen et al. (1987a). The proximal aorta is an area susceptible to the development of diet-induced atherosclerosis in the mouse. The quantitative assay utilized in these studies is dependent on the determination of the area of lipid-staining regions in four to five separate aortic sections from animals which have been fed atherogenic diets for 3–6 months. The results of our studies in the AI transgenic animals compared to controls are illustrated in Fig. 4. When placed on high fat diets and compared to their nontransgenic litter mates, the C57BL/6 transgenic mice containing and expressing the human apoAI transgene are highly protected from the development of diet-induced atherosclerosis (Rubin et al. 1991). We found that the AI transgenic mice had a much smaller fatty streak lesion area per section on the atherogenic

                                    Edward Rubin and Joshua Schultz

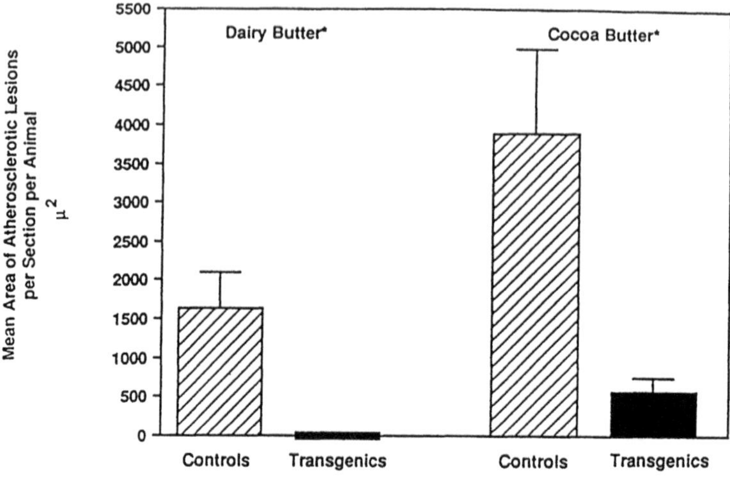

Fig. 4. A quantitative assessment of atherogenesis in transgenic and control mice fed two different high fat (15 %) and high cholesterol (1.0 %–1.25 %) diets for 14–18 weeks. The area of lipid staining material per section per animal was assessed for over 20 animals in each group. *Significant difference between transgenic and control mice at *p*

diets. Expression of the human apoAI gene resulted in complete protection from the development of fatty streak lesions in the transgenic animals on the dairy butter high fat diet [containing 15 % fat (the primary source being dairy butter fat), 1 % cholesterol, 0.5 % sodium choleate and 20 % casein]. On the more atherogenic cocoa butter diet [15 % fat (the primary source being cocoa butter), 1.25 % cholesterol, 0.5 % sodium choleate and 7.5 % casein] an approximate sevenfold reduction in lesion area was observed.

Our results from these studies indicate, (1) the importance of apoAI in determining the level and particle size of HDL, (2) the existence of a post-transcriptional mechanism which alters the plasma level of the endogenous mouse apoAI, and (3) that high plasma concentrations of human apoAI protects C57BL/6 mice from developing atherosclerosis. The association between high apoAI/HDL levels and protection from atherosclerosis remains an unresolved issue in humans. HDL's antiatherogenic or protective role is widely believed to be due to its ability to remove cholesterol from the circulation and promote its degradation via the "reverse cholesterol transport" pathway (Fielding and Fielding 1982). According to this model, HDL is thought to be responsible for scavenging cholesterol from peripheral tissue. Cholesterol in the cell membrane is esterified by LCAT in the presence of HDL and is then transferred to other lipoproteins or degraded into bile acids and excreted via the intestines. This model is supported by epidemiological data as well as by in vitro studies in which HDL has been shown to bind to various cells and promote cholesterol efflux (Barbaras et al. 1987). Our studies demonstrate that high human apoAI and HDL concentrations in mice directly inhibit a polygenic form of atherosclerosis in this animal. These results support the hypothesis that apoAI and HDL may have direct antiatherogenic effects and indicate that therapeutic interventions which raise the plasma levels of these factors may decrease the risk of atherosclerosis in humans.

2.4 Transgenic Mice Expressing Human ApoAI and Human ApoAII

In conjunction with these human apoAI studies, we also characterized the effect of high level expression of the other major HDL-associated apolipoprotein, apoAII. Transgenic mice expressing human apoAII (AII transgenic mice), and both human apoAI and human apoAII (AI/AII transgenic mice) were produced in the C67BL/6 strain. Human apoAII mRNA is expressed exclusively in the livers of AII transgenic animals and the protein exists as a dimer, as it does in humans. Contrary to what was observed in the human AI transgenic mice, increases in plasma apoAII of up to twofold had little effect on the endogenous apoAI and apoAII plasma levels or on the HDL concentrations of AII transgenic mice. The AII transgenic mice contain the major HDL size population present in control C57BL/6 mice and, in addition, have a smaller sized population of HDL particles. AI/AII transgenic mice had HDL concentrations similar to that of the AI transgenic mice, further supporting a primary and dominant role for apoAI in determining HDL concentration. HDL from the AI/AII transgenic mice displayed a unique size distribution when compared with either AI or AII transgenic mice and contain particles with both human apoAI and human apoAII. These results suggest that human apoAII in the plasma of transgenic mice has little effect on HDL levels but does participate in determining HDL size, especially when associated with human apoAI.

Size distribution profiles of HDL from the AI and AI/AII transgenic mice mimic the size distributions of the human Lp(AI w/o AII) and Lp(AI w AII) subpopulations, respectively. It has been hypothesized that human plasma Lp(AI w AII) and Lp(AI w/o AII) have different physiological properties with regard to both the ability of these particles to participate in reverse cholesterol transport and the role they play in atherosclerosis (Fielding, and Fielding 1981 and 1982; Barbaras et al. 1987; Puchois et al. 1987; Nichols et al. 1987). The similarities between Lp(AI w AII) and Lp(AI w/o AII) in humans and HDL in the AI and AI/AII transgenic mice have led us to investigate the effects that these HDL subpopulations have on the susceptibility to diet-induced atherosclerosis. In these studies, transgenic mice (AI and AI/AII) with similar HDL levels but different apolipoprotein-specific HDL populations are being examined to investigate the antiatherogenic properties of HDL subclasses containing AI with AII and AI without AII.

In summary, to gain a better understanding of the function of apoAI and apoAII and to determine what effect different plasma concentrations of these apolipoproteins have on HDL and atherosclerosis, transgenic mice were produced expressing human apoAI, apoAII, and both apoAI and apoAII. High levels of expression of the human apoAI with or without human apoAII is associated with a twofold increase in HDL cholesterol, a major decrease ($\sim 90\,\%$) in endogenous murine apoAI and a substantial decrease ($\sim 40\,\%$) in the endogenous murine apoAII plasma concentrations. Studies have indicated that the decrease in murine apoAI occurs posttranscriptionally (Rubin et al. 1991) and that the catabolism of human apoAI and murine apoAI are identical in transgenic mice (Walsh et al. 1989). Transgenic mice with high plasma levels of apoAI and HDL are significantly protected from the development of atherosclerotic fatty streak lesions. In contrast to what was found in human AI transgenic mice, high level expression of the human apoAII transgene does not significantly affect the plasma concentrations of mouse apoAI, apoAII, or HDL cholesterol. The HDL particle size distribution, however, is altered in both the AI and AII transgenic mice. Evidence from AI/AII transgenic mice further supports a role for apoAI in determining structure and level of HDL, while apoAII plays mainly a structural role.

References

Barbaras R, Puchois P, Fruchart JC (1987) Cholesterol efflux from cultured adipose cells is mediated by LpA_I particles but not LpA_IA_{II} particles. Biochem Biophys Res Comm 42(1):63–69

Blanche PJ, Gong EL, Forte TM, Nichols AV (1981) Characterization of human high-density lipoproteins by gradient gel electrophoresis. Biochim Biophys Acta 665:408–19

Cheung MC, Albers JJ (1984) Characterization of lipoprotein particles isolated by immunoaffinity chromatography: Particles containing A-I and A-II and particles containing A-I but no A-II. J Biol Chem 259:12201–12209

Cheung MC, Wolf AC, Lum KD, Tollefson JH, Albers JJ (1986) Distribution and localization of lecithin: Cholesterol acyltransferase and cholesterol ester activity in A-I-containing lipoproteins. J Lipid Res 27:1135–1144

Cheung MC, Nichols AV, Blanche PJ, Gong EL, Franceschini G, Sirtori CR (1988) Characterization of A-I-containing lipoproteins in subjects with A-I Milano variant. Biochim Biophys Acta 960:73–82

Eggerman TL, Hoeg JM, Meng MS, Tombragel A, Bojanovski D, Brewer HB Jr (1991) Differential tissue-specific expression of human apoA-I and apoA-II. J Lipid Res 32:821–828

Fielding CJ, Fielding PE (1981) Evidence for a lipoprotein carrier in human plasma catalyzing sterol efflux from cultured fibroblasts and its relationship to Lecithin: cholesterol acyltransferase. Proc Natl Acad Sci USA 78:3911–3914

Fielding CJ, Fielding PE (1982) Cholesterol transport between cells and body fluids. Role of plasma lipoproteins and the plasma cholesterol esterification system. Med Clin N Am 66: 363–373

Frager G, Wiklund O, Olofsson SO, Norfelt P, Wilhelmson L, Bondjers G (1979) Serum apolipoprotein levels in relation to acute myocardial infarction and its risk factors, determination of polypeptide AII. Artery 6:188–204

Frohlich JJ, Pritchard PH (1989) The clinical significance of serum high density lipoproteins. Clin Biochem 22:417–423

Glueck M, Costa E, Fullert R, Sielski J, Steinen P (1976) Longevity syndromes: Familial hyperalphalipoproteinemia. J Lab Clin Med 88:941–944

Gofman J, Jones HB, Lindgren FT, Lyon TP, Elliott HA, Strisower B (1950) Blood lipids and human atherosclerosis. Circulation 2:161–178

Haddad IA, Ordovas JM, Fitzpatrick T, Karathanasis S (1986) Linkage, evolution and expression of the rat apolipoprotein AI, CIII, and AIV genes. J Biol Chem 261:13268–13277

Karathanasis SK (1985) Apolipoprotein multigene family: tandem organization of human apolipoprotein AI-CIII and A-IV genes. Proc Natl Acad Sci USA 82:6374–6378

Lackner KJ, Law SW, Brewer HB Jr, Sakaguchi AY, Naylor SL (1984) The human apolipoprotein A-II gene is located on chromosome 1. Biochem Biopys Res Commun 122:877–883

LeBoeuf RC, Doolittle MH, Montcalm A, Martin DC, Reue K, Lusis AJ (1990) Phenotypic characterization of the Ath-1 gene controlling high density lipoprotein levels and susceptibility to atherosclerosis. J Lip Res 31:91–101

Lusis AJ, Taylor BA, Wangenstein RW, LeBoeuf RC (1983) Genetic control of lipid transport in mice. II. Genes controlling structure of high density lipoproteins. J Biol Chem 258(8): 5071–5078

Maciejko JJ, Holmes DR, Kottke BA, Zinsmeisten AR, Dinh DM, Mao SJT (1983) Apolipoprotein AI as marker of angiographically assessed coronary artery disease. N Engl J Med 309:385–389

Miller JC, Barth RK, Shaw PH, Elliott RW, Hastie ND (1983) Proc Natl Acad Sci USA 80:1511–1515

Miller NE (1987) Associations of high-density lipoprotein subclasses and apolipoproteins with ischemic heart disease and coronary atherosclerosis. Am Heart J 113:589–597

Nichols AV, Gong EL, Blanche PJ, Forte TM, Shore VG (1987) Pathways in the formation of human plasma high density lipoprotein subpopulations containing apolipoprotein A-I without apolipoprotein A–II. J Lipid Res 28: 719–732

Nichols AV, Cheung MC, Blanche PJ, Gong EL, Francheschini G, Sirtori CR (1989) Apolipoprotein-specific high density lipoprotein populations in plasma of carriers of the apolipoprotein AI-Milano. In: Sirtori CR, Francheschini G, Brewer HB Jr, Assmann G (eds) Human Apolipoprotein Mutants: From Gene Structure to Phenotypic Expression. Plenum Press, New York, pp 67–73

Paigen B, Morrow A, Brandon C, Mitchell D, Homles P (1985) Variation in susceptibility to atherosclerosis among inbred strains of mice. Atherosclerosis 57:65–74

Paigen B, Homles P, Mitchell D, Albee D (1987a) Comparison of atherosclerotic lesions and HDL-lipid levels in male, female, and testosterone-treated female mice from strains C57BL/6, BALB/c, and C3H. Atherosclerosis 64:215–221

Paigen B, Mitchell D, Reue K, Morrow A, Lusis AJ, LeBoeuf RC (1987b) Ath-1, a gene determining atherosclerosis susceptibility and high density lipoprotein levels in mice. Proc Natl Acad Sci USA 84:3763–3767

Paigen B, Nesbitt MN, Mitchell D, Albee D, LeBoeuf RC (1989) Ath-2, a second gene determining atherosclerosis susceptibility and high density lipoprotein levels in mice. Genetics 122:163–168

Paigen B, Ishida BY, Verstuyft J, Winters RB, Albee D (1990) Atherosclerosis susceptibility differences among progenitors of recombinant inbred strains of mice. Arteriosclerosis 10(2):316–323

Puchois P, Kandoussi A, Fievet P, Fourrier JL, Bertrand M, Koren E, Fruchart JC (1987) Apolipoprotein A-I containing lipoproteins in coronary artery disease. Atherosclerosis 68:35–40

Roberts A, Thompson JS (1976) Inbred mice and their hybrids as an animal model for atherosclerosis research. In: Day CE (ed) Atherosclerosis Drug Discovery, Plenum Press, NY, pp 313–327

Rubin EM, Ishida BY, Clift SM, Krauss RM (1991a) Expression of human apolipoprotein A-I in transgenic mice results in reduced plasma levels of murine apolipoprotein A-I and the appearance of two new high density lipoprotein size subclasses. Proc Natl Acad Sci USA 88: 434–438

Rubin EM, Krauss RM, Spangler EA, Verstuyft JG, Clift SM (1991b) Inhibition of early atherogenesis in transgenic mice by human apolipoprotein A-I. Nature 353: 265–267

Schaefer EJ, Heaton WH, Wetzel MG, Brewer HB Jr (1982) Plasma apolipoprotein AI absence associated with a marked reduction of high density lipoproteins and premature coronary artery disease. Arteriosclerosis 2:16–26

Stewart-Phillips JL, Lough J (1991) Pathology of atherosclerosis in cholesterol-fed, susceptible mice. Atherosclerosis 90:211–218

Stewart-Phillips JL, Lough J, Skamene E (1988) Genetically determined susceptibility and resistance to diet-induced atherosclerosis in inbred strains of mice. J Lab Clin Med 112:36–42

Stewart-Phillips JL, Lough J, Skomene E (1989) Ath-3 a new gene for atherosclerosis in mice. Clin Invest Med 12, 121–126

3 The PrP-less Mouse: A Tool for Prion Research

Charles Weissmann, Hansruedi Büeler, Marek Fischer,
and Michel Aguet

The nature of the agent causing transmissible spongiform encephalopathies (TSE), such as scrapie or bovine spongiform encephalopathy in animals or Creutzfeldt-Jakob disease (CJD) and Gerstmann-Sträussler-Scheinker disease (GSS) in man, is still controversial (for recent reviews, see Prusiner 1991; Weissmann 1991a; Kimberlin 1990; Aiken and Marsh 1990; Bruce and Fraser 1991; Rohwer 1991). In this article we will review the current hypotheses regarding the pathogenesis of this class of diseases and describe an approach designed to test critically the so-called "protein only" hypothesis.

3.1 Transmissible Spongiform Encephalopathies

The overall properties of the infectious agents of TSE's, which has been designated as "prion" (Prusiner 1982), differ from those of any known virus or viroid (Gordon 1946; Pattison 1965; Prusiner 1982; Brown et al. 1990). Prusiner has suggested that the prion is devoid of nucleic acid and identical with PrP^{Sc}, a modified form of PrP^C (the "protein only" hypotheses; Prusiner 1989). PrP^C is a normal host protein (Oesch et al. 1985; Chesebro et al. 1985; Hope et al. 1986) en-

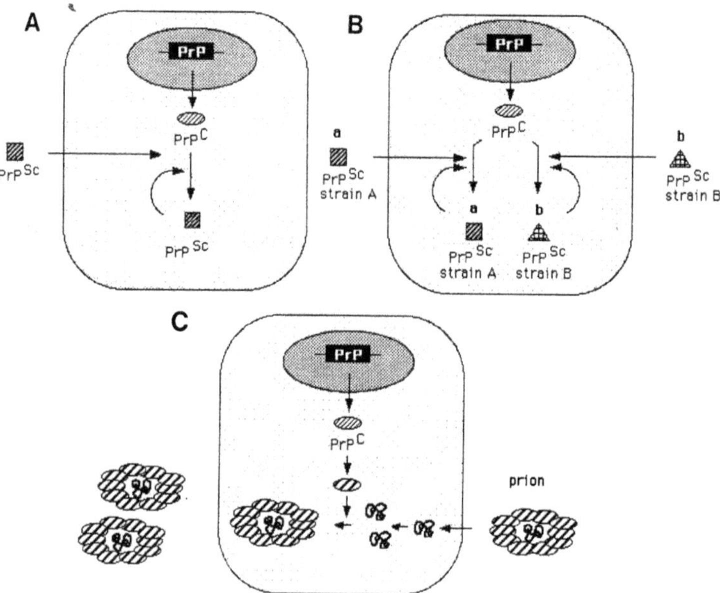

Fig. 1A–C. Models for the propagation of the scrapie agent (prion). **A,B** The "protein only" model assumes that the prion is identical with PrP^{Sc}. **A** Exogenous prions cause the conversion of the normal cellular protein PrP^C and PrP^{Sc}. **B** Many different strains of prions are known. Because there is only one *Prn-p* gene, each strain of prion must impose its particular strain specific structure (be it chemical or conformational) on the single species of PrP^C or its precursor (**C**). The "virino hypothesis" assumes that the infectious agent consists of a nucleic acid associated with or packaged in PrP^{Sc}. The "scrapie-specific nucleic acid" is replicated in the cell and recruits PrP^C into association with it. Strain specificity would by mediated by the nucleic acid

coded within a single exon of a single-copy gene (Basler et al. 1986) and is found predominantly on the surface of neurons, attached by a glycoinositol phospholipid anchor (Prusiner 1989; Prusiner and DeArmond 1990; Prusiner 1991; Stahl et al. 1987), but also in a variety of other tissues, both in the embryonic and the adult mouse (Hope and Manson 1992; Bendheim et al. 1992).

PrP^{Sc} is defined as a protease-resistant form of PrP^{C} which readily aggregates after treatment with detergents and protease (Prusiner et al. 1982; Prusiner et al. 1983; Oesch et al. 1985; McKinley et al. 1991). It accumulates intracellularly in cytoplasmic vesicles (Taraboulos et al. 1990; McKinley et al. 1990) and is the major component of the extracellular amyloid plaques characteristic for prion diseases. No chemical differences have so far been detected between PrP^{Sc} and PrP^{C} (Turk et al. 1988; Prusiner 1991; Stahl, Baldwin and Prusiner, personal communication).

Prusiner proposed that PrP^{Sc}, when introduced into a normal cell, causes the conversion of PrP^{C} or its precursor into PrP^{Sc} (Oesch et al. 1985; Oesch et al. 1988; Prusiner et al. 1990; Prusiner 1991; Bolton and Bendheim 1988) (Fig. 1a). The nature of the conversion is unknown and could be due to a chemical or conformational modification, during or after its synthesis. However, the existence of many different strains of scrapie which can be propagated in one and the same inbred mouse line and the apparent mutability of the agent (Kimberlin 1990; Aiken and Marsh 1990; Bruce and Fraser 1991) are cited in support of the virino hypothesis (Fig. 1c). This hypothesis holds that the infectious agent consists of a nucleic acid genome and the host-derived PrP, which is recruited as some sort of coat (Oesch et al. 1985; Dickinson and Outram 1988), but no evidence for such a nucleic acid has yet been adduced (Aiken and Marsh 1990; Meyer et al. 1991; Oesch et al. 1988; Kellings et al. 1992).

Several lines of evidence argue that the prion consists entirely or at least in part of PrP^{Sc}:

1. Scrapie infectivity is associated with Prp^{Sc}. purification of scrapie infectivity results in a preparation highly enriched with regard to PrP^{Sc} (Bolton et al. 1982; Diringer et al. 1983; Prusiner et al. 1982), Conversely, purification of PrP^{Sc} by affinity chromatography on an

anti-PrP antibody column leads to enrichment of infectivity (Gabizon et al. 1988).

2. A nucleic acid larger than about 100 nucleotides is not essential for infectivity of scrapie prion preparations. This claim is based on (a) the unusually small target size of scrapie infectivity for UV and ionizing radiation (Alper et al. 1967; Latarjet et al. 1970; Bellinger-Kawahara et al. 1988), (b) the low ratio of nucleic acids to infectious units in highly purified prion preparations (Kellings et al. 1992) and the failure to find scrapie-specific nucleic acid in prion preparations or scrapie-infected brain tissue (Aiken and Marsh 1990; Oesch et al. 1988; Diedrich et al. 1987), and (c) resistance of infectivity to treatment with agents modifying or damaging nucleic acids (Prusiner 1982). All together, these data suggest that a nucleic acid of more than 50–100 nucleotides is not required for infectivity (but see Sklaviadis et al. 1990 for a different conclusion).

3. The susceptibility of a host to scrapie infection is codetermined by the prion inoculum and the Prn-p gene. The significance of the host PrP genotype for the susceptibility to scrapie infection and the course of the disease is revealed by two sets of findings. First, the incubation time for one and the same prion isolate may be different in distinct mouse strains and is determined predominantly by the *Sinc* (Dickinson et al. 1968; Bruce and Dickinson 1987) or *Prn-i* gene (Carlson et al. 1968; Hunter et al. 1987), which is very closely linked to or coincident with *Prn-p* – the gene encoding PrP (Carlson et al. 1986; Hunter et al. 1987; Carlson et al. 1988; Carlson et al. 1989; Race et al. 1990). Second, when prions are transmitted from one animal species to another, disease often develops only after a very long incubation period, if at all; however, upon serial passaging in the new species, the incubation time may decrease dramatically and then stabilize. This so-called species barrier (Pattison 1966) can be overcome by introducing into the recipient host the PrP transgene from the prion dunor (Scott et al. 1989; Prusiner et al. 1990). Moreover, prion preparations from mice carrying hamster PrP-transgenes and inoculated with hamster scrapie prions are highly infectious to the hamster but not to the mouse. The same transgenic mouse strain, infected with mouse-derived prions, yields preprations highly infectious for mice but not for hamsters (Prusiner et al. 1990). Within the framework of the "protein only" hypo-

thesis this means that hamster PrP^C, but not murine PrP^C, is a suitable substrate for conversion to hamster PrP^{Sc} by hamster prions and vice versa.

4. Hereditary forms of spongiform encephalopathies are linked to mutations of the Prn-p gene. The human prion diseases, CJD and GSS, are very rare in the overall population, but also occur as a familiar form (Gibbs et al. 1968; Gajdusek 1977; Masters et al. 1981b; Masters et al. 1981a). Hsiao et al. (1989) found that in the two apparently unrelated GSS families the disease is tightly linked to a proline-to-leucine change in codon 102 of one of the alleles of the PrP gene. Subsequently, other GSS and CJD families were identified which carry the 102 mutation or one of a number of other mutations in the PrP gene (for a review see Baker and Ridley 1992). Prusiner (1989, 1991) proposed that the mutations allow spontaneous conversion of PrP^C into PrP^{Sc} with a frequency sufficient to allow the disease to be expressed within the lifetime of the individual. Sporadic CJD and GSS would be attributable to a somatic mutation in the PrP gene or to a rare instance of spontaneous conversion of PrP^C into PrP^{Sc}.

Hsiao et al. (1990) showed that mice carrying a murine PrP transgene with the pro→leu mutation corresponding to the human GSS mutation at position 102 spontaneously come down with a lethal scrapie-like disease. However, PrP^{Sc} was not detected and it has not yet been definitively determined whether or not the brains of these animals contain infectious prions.

The experimental data outlined above argue persuasively that the prion is composed partly or entirely of a PrP isoform (either PrP^{Sc} or a subfraction of it) and that protein-encoding nucleic acid is not an essential component.

Prusiner proposed that PrP^{Sc}, when introduced into a normal cell, causes the conversion of PrP^C or its precursor into PrP^{Sc} (Oesch et al. 1985; Oesch et al. 1988; Prusiner et al. 1990; Prusiner 1991; Bolton and Bendheim 1988). Because no chemical differences between PrP^C and PrP^{Sc} have been detected, Prusiner postulated a difference in the conformation of the two species. In Fig. 2a it is suggested that a molecule of PrP^{Sc} binds to PrP^C and thereby imposes its conformation upon it. The species barrier is explained by the assumption that heterologous

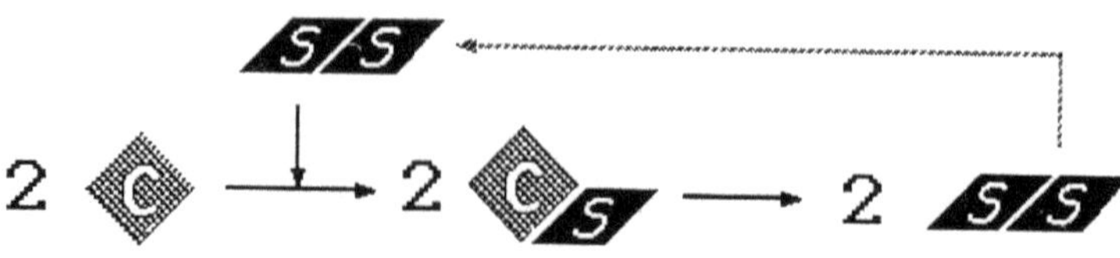

Fig. 2. Model for the catalyzed conformational conversion of PrP^C to an infectious PrP form. Scheme based on a proposal of Prusiner (Prusiner et al. 1990)

PrP species interact poorly and/or that the conversion only occurs rarely. The Gerstmann-Sträussler type mutations would allow spontaneous, albeit very rare, conversion events, yielding PrP^{Sc} that can then act catalytically.

The finding that there are many distinct strains of scrapie prions which can be propagated in one and the same mouse strain (homozygous with regard to its Prn-p gene) is not readily explained by the "protein only" hypothesis (for a review, see Brucer and Fraser 1991) because it implies that an incoming PrP^{Sc} strain can convert one and the same PrP precursor into a likeness of itself, and that this can happen for several if not many different strains.

Two subsidiary hypotheses have been suggested to circumvent this difficulty. The "unified theory" (Weissmann 1991b) proposes that PrP^{Sc} is associated with a small nucleic acid which is not required for infectivity but determines the characteristic phenotype of the strain. This nucleic acid would be replicated by host cell enzymes and then associate with newly formed PrP^{Sc}, leading to preservation of the prion's phenotype. The "targeting theory" (K.H. Meyer, personal communication 1991; Hecker et al. 1992) proposes that PrP^{Sc} carries a variable modification, for example, carbohydrate residues, which target it to a specific subset of cells. These cells would impart the same modification to the newly formed PrP^{Sc} molecules. Different strains would thus be targeted to different subsets of cells and retain their specific modification. This hypotheses is supported by the observation that two different hamster prion strains (Hecker et al. 1992) or mouse prion strains (Manson et al. 1992) give rise to different patterns of PrP^{Sc} deposition in the brain.

3.2 Generation of Mice Devoid of PrP^C

The "protein only" hypothesis predicts that in the absence of PrP^C, mice should be resistant to scrapie infection, both with regard to symptoms and to propagation of the infectious agent. We therefore undertook to generate mice with disrupted *prn-p* alleles (Büeler et al. 1992), hoping that even if such mice were not viable, it might at least be possible to generate neuronal tissue cultures which might be tested for infectability.

3.2.1 Generation and Properties of Prn-p$^{0/0}$ Mice

We disrupted one *Prn-p* allele of murine embryonic stem (ES) cells by homologous recombination with a 4.8-kb DNA fragment in which codons 4 to 187 of the 254-codon open reading frame were replaced by a neomycin phosphotransferase (*neo*) gene under the control of the HSV TK promoter (Fig. 3). In the resulting construction the first 3 *Prn-p* codons, the *neo* coding sequence and the residual 67 *Prn-p* codons were fused in frame, with one nonsense codon interposed between the initial *Prn-p* codons and the *neo* sequence and two nonsense codons between the latter and the residual *Prn-p* sequence (Fig. 3D).

Blastocysts were injected with cells carrying the disrupted *Prn-p* gene and implanted into foster mothers. Chimeric males were mated with wild-type mice, and offspring carrying the disrupted gene were identified by polymerase chain reaction (PCR) analysis. *Prn-p$^{0/+}$* heterozygotes were mated and 176 superficially indistinguishable offspring analyzed by PCR. Of these, 24% were homozygous for the disrupted *Prn-p* gene.

3.2.2 Molecular Genetic Characterization

As shown by northern analysis, normal PrP mRNA was not detectable in brain from *Prn-p$^{0/0}$* homozygotes; however, substantial quantities of a fused mRNA containing the *neo* and the residual *Prn-p* sequence were present. Western analysis of brain proteins showed that a set of

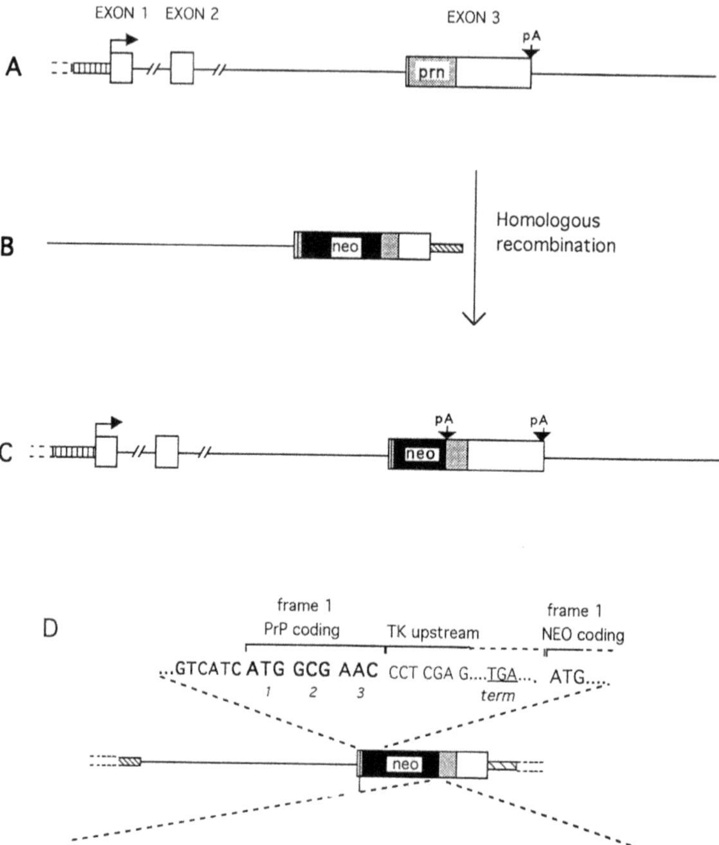

Fig. 3. A Map of the murine *Prn-p* gene (Westaway et al. 1987). **B** The targeting vector was constructed by replacing 552 bp of the *Prn-p* coding region (extending from position 10 to 562) by a 1.1-kb cassette containing the TK promoter followed by the *neo* gene. **C** Map of the disrupted *Prn-p* gene. **D** The first 3 *Prn-p* codons, the *neo* coding sequence and the residual 67 *Prn-p* codons were fused in frame, with one nonsense codon interposed between the initial *Prn-p* codons and the *neo* sequence and two nonsense codons between the latter and the residual *Prn-p* sequence

bands present in wild-type samples was absent in $Prn-p^{0/0}$ samples and present at about half the level in $Prn-p^{0/+}$ samples.

3.2.3 Physical Characterization

No gross abnormalities were noted, as judged by the size, weight and appearance of the brain, skeletal muscle, and visceral organs in the homozygous $Prn-p^{0/0}$ mice. The histology of the brain was the same in wild-type and homozygous $Prn-p^{0/0}$ mice. Skeletal muscle was also normal, as judged by histochemical analysis of fiber types and distribution of sarcoplasmic reticulum. Homozygous $Prn-p^{0/0}$ mice are fertile and normal progeny result from homozygous $Prn-p^{0/0}$ breeding pairs. No spontaneous deaths of homozygotes were recorded during the 15-month period of observation.

3.2.4 Immunological Characterization

It has been reported that PrP^C is expressed on the surface of B and T lymphocytes and that it participates in lymphocyte activation (Cashman et al. 1990). We therefore compared some immunological parameters of thymocytes and splenocytes of 6-week-old $Prn-p^{+/+}$ and $Prn-p^{0/0}$ mice. Disruption of the $Prn-p$ gene had no detectable effect on the level of cell surface IgM, CD3, CD4/8, or MHC class I and class II antigens (Table 1), indicating that PrP^C is not essential for the normal maturation of the lymphocyte subsets. No significant difference in the response of splenocytes from $Prn-p^{0/0}$ and $Prn-p^{+/+}$ mice to activation by concanavalin A was detected (Table 2).

3.2.5 Behavior

Because PrP^C is a predominantly neuronal protein and present in a high proportion of hippocampal neurons, the learning ability of $Prn-p^{0/0}$ and $Prn-p^{+/+}$ and $Prn-p^{0/+}$ mice, all derived from the mating of the first generation of heterozygotes, was compared using three tests. In the *swimming navigation,* or *swim test* (Morris 1984), the animal is

Table 1. FACS analysis of splenocytes and thymocytes of wild-type and PRP$^{0/0}$ mice

Antigen	Mean relative fluorescence (percent of cells)			
	Splenocytes Wild type	PrP$^{0/0}$	Thymocytes Wild type	PrP$^{0/0}$
CD3	15.44 (28.7%)	15.07 (36.4%)	5.66 (44.5%)	7.37 (44.6%)
MHC I	9.79 (98.8%)	10.68 (98.4%)	7.24 (8.7%)	7.32 (7.3%)
MCH II	10.96 (58.3%)	10.30 (60,9%)	3.05 (12.5%)	2.82 (7.3%)
IgM	11.27 (57.7%)	11.20 (58.8%)	3.40 (0.6%)	3.60 (0.7%)
CD4	10.09 (14.9%)	11.46 (19.2%)	9.43 (7.8%)	8.90 (12.7%)
CD8	0.18 (6.9%)	0.19 (9.9%)	0.60 (2.9%)	0.61 (3.9%)
CD4/CD8 (ratio)	2.16	1.94	2.96	3.26

Single cell suspensions from thymus or spleen of 6-week-old mice were adjusted to 2×10^6 cells/100 µl and reacted with primary antibodies for 30 min at 4C in BSS (0.14 M NaCl, 1 mM CaCl$_2$, 5.4 mM KCl, 0.8 mM MgSo$_4$, 0.3 mM Na$_2$HPO$_4$, pH 6.9) plus 2% fetal calf serum and 0.1% NaN$_3$. The cells were washed by centrifugation with BSS and incubated where necessary with secondary antibody. After a further washing step, cell-associated fluorescence was quantified in a EPICS Profile fluorescence activated cell sorter (Coulter Corp., Florida). Primary antibodies used were the hybridoma supernatants KT3 (rat anti-CD3 antibody), K7-309 (mouse anti-MHC I, H2K^b, antibody; Hämmerling et al. 1982), and K25-137.1 (mouse anti-MHC II antibody; Koch et al. 1982), FITC-conjugated rat antibodies specific for IgM and CD8 (Becton-Dickinson), as well as PE-conjugated rat antibody against CD4 (Becton-Dickinson). Secondary antibodies were FITC-conjugated goat anti-mouse IgG2a (Southern Biotechnology Associates, Cat. # 1080-02) or goat anti-rat IgG (Tago Inc., Cat. # 6720), respectively.

placed in a pool and must learn to find a submerged platform with the aid of extramaze visual cues. Swimming navigation has high cognitive demands, is severely impaired after hippocampal lesions, and reveals behavioral correlates of genetically determined morphological and physiological differences in the intact hippocampus. There were no significant group differences in learning to find the submerged platform. The *Y-maze discrimination* test (Lipp and Van der Loos 1991) assesses the ability of mice to avoid punishment by means of a direc-

Table 2. Stimulation of splenocytes by concanavalin A

	Con A (mg//l)	^{3}H-thymidine incorporation cpm x10^{-3} (stimulation index)			
		PrP$^{+/+}$		PrP$^{0/0}$	
Day 3	0	4 ± 0.6	–	9 ± 1	–
	1	143 ± 5	(36)	125 ± 4	(14)
	10	163 ± 9	(41)	124 ± 6	(14)
Day 4	0	4 ± 0.5	(1)	11 ± 2	(1)
	1	39 ± 9	(10)	42 ± 4	(4)
	10	187 ± 7	(47)	123 ± 12	(11)

Splenocytes were isolated from PrP$^{0/0}$ or Prp$^{+/+}$ mice and grown in 96-well plates ($2x10^5$ cells/well) in DMEM with nonessential amino acids (Gibco) containing the concentration of concanavalin A indicated. After 3 and 4 days, respectively, proliferation of splenocytes was measured by adding 0.5 µC ^{3}H-thymidine (80 Ci/mmol) to each well 5 h before harvesting and measuring acid insoluble radioactivity. The values given are the means of quadruplicate measurements on four mice for each point the standard error. The stimulation index is the ratio of radioactivity incorporated in the presence to that in the absence of concanavalin A

tional decision (go left or right) based on visual and vibrissotactile cues presented randomly either in the left or right arm of the maze. Wild types, hetero- and homozygotes showed no significant differences in discrimination learning. The *two-way avoidance (shuttlebox)* test (Anisman 1978) is a sensitive indicator for hippocampal malfunction as well as for many other behavioral abnormalities. There was no statistically significant difference between the different groups.

The results of the behavioral tests showed that *Prn-p$^{0/0}$* and *Prn-p$^{0/+}$* mice were not impaired in learning ability, also in difficult tasks likely to reveal even minor brain damage.

3.3 Implications and Outlook

3.3.1 PrP-less Mice Have No Apparent Phenotype

It is interesting that a protein expressed in many areas of the brain and in other tissues, particularly during embryonic development, in all species of mammals examined and in at least one bird, and which shows a rapid turnover is expendable without a detrimental effect. In lower eukaryotes, homozygous gene disruptions that fail to engender phenotypic changes are quite frequent; it has been estimated that in *Saccharomyces cerevisiae* almost half of gene disruptions fail to display an obvious phenotype (Goebl and Petes 1986). Many examples have been described for *Caenorhabditis elegans* (Ferguson and Horvitz 1989) and some for *Drosophila* (Elkins et al. 1990). One explanation for the apparent expendability of a gene product is that the resulting defect only becomes apparent in advanced age or is so subtle that a selective disadvantage may emerge only after many generations, perhaps under stressful natural conditions. Such functional defects might only become detectable by targeted assays, when one knows that to look for, as in the case of HPRT null mice (Hooper et al. 1987) $\beta2$ microglobulin-deficient (Zijlstra et al. 1990; Koller et al. 1990) or IL-2-deficient mice (Schorle et al. 1991). Another possibility is that the function of the missing protein within the cell is assumed by related or different protein(s), or that the function is redundant at the organismic level. In *Drosophila* neither protein null mutations of fasciclin I, a GPI-linked neuronal cell adhesion molecule, nor of Abelson cytoplasmic tyrosine kinase lead to gross defects, but double mutants show a clear defect in growth cone guidance (Elkins et al. 1990). En-2-deficient-mice, while possessing a smaller cerebellum with an altered pattern of folding, show no functional abnormalities, perhaps because of functional redundancy due to the structurally related En-1 gene (Joyner et al. 1991). Finally, it is conceivable that in some cases a protein may have been required earlier in evolution, but no longer serves any function, and that it has been conserved not by selective pressure but because of evolutionary inertia.

3.3.2 Implications for Prion Research

So far, it has been unclear whether the pathology of scrapie is due to the depletion of normal PrP^C or to the accumulation of PrP^{Sc} in infected neurons. The fact that mice can live normally for at least 15 months without expressing any PrP^C argues against the "loss-of-function" hypothesis.

The possibility of raising *Prn-p^{0/0}* mice allows us to determine whether mice devoid of PrP^C, after infection with scrapie, (a) show scrapie symptoms and (b) allow the multiplication of prions. If the mice are deficient in regard to either or both of these properties, it should be possible to delineate, by reverse genetics, which domains of PrP are essential for the required functions.

3.3.3 Possible Practical Applications

Should mice devoid of PrP^C indeed be resistant to scrapie infection, and if the expendability of these genes is a general phenomenon, it might be feasible to raise livestock impervious to the disease. By the same token, therapy aimed at diminishing the synthesis of PrP^C (for example, anti-sense oligonucleotides in conjunction with an agent permitting transfer across the blood–brain barrier, or specific inhibition of PrP gene transcription) might provide a rational approach to retard and mitigate disease progression in man.

Acknowledgements. This work was supported by the Erziehungsdirektion of the Kanton of Zürich and grants of the Schweizerische Nationalfonds to C.W. We thank Dr. S. Prusiner for advice and discussions.

References

Aiken JM, Marsh RF (1990) The search for scrapie agent nucleic acid. Microbiol Ref 54: 242–246

Alper T, Cramp WA, Haig DA, Clarke MC (1967) Does the agent of scrapie replicate without nucleic acid. Nature 214: 764–766

Anisman H (1978) In: Anisman H, Bignami G (eds) The psychopharmacology of aversively motivated behavior. Plenum Press, New York, pp 1–62

Baker HF, Ridley RM (1992) The genetics and transmissibility of human spongiform encephalopathy. Neurodegeneration 1:3–16

Basler K, Oesch B, Scott M, Westaway D, Wälchli M, Groth DF, McKinley MP, Prusiner SB, and Weissmann C (1986) Scrapie and cellular PrP isoforms are encoded by the same chromosomal gene. Cell 46:417–428

Bellinger-Kawahara CG, Kempner E, Groth D, Gabizon R, and Prusinger SB (1988) Scrabie prion liposomes and rods exhibit target sizes of 55,000 Da. Virology 164:537–541

Bendheim PE, Brown HR, Rudelli RC, Scala LJ, Goller NL, Wen GY, Kascsak RJ, Cashman NR, Bolton DC (1992) Nearly ubiquitous tissue distribution of the scrapie agent precursor protein. Neurology 42:149–156

Bolton DC, Bendheim PE (1988) In: Bock G, Marsh J (eds) Novel Infectious Agents and the Central Nervous System. John Wiley & Sons, Chichester, pp 164–177

Bolton DC, McKinley MP, Prusiner SB (1982) Identification of a protein that purifies with the scrapie prion. Science 218:1309–1311

Brown P, Liberski PP, Wolff A, Gajdusek DC (1990) Resistance of scrapie infectivity to steam autoclaving after formaldehyde fixation and limited survival after ashing at 360 degrees C: practical and theoretical implications. J Infect Dis 161:467–472

Bruce ME, Dickinson AG (1987) Biological evidence that scrapie agents has an independent genome. J Gen Virol 68:79–89

Bruce ME, Fraser H (1991) Scrapie strain variation and its implications. Curr Top Microbiol Immunol 172:125–138

Büeler H, Fischer M, Lang Y, Bluethmann H, Lipp HP, DeArmond SJ, Prusiner SB, Aguet M, Weissmann C (1992) Normal development and behaviour of mice lacking the neuronal cell-surface PrP protein (see comments). Nature 356:577–582

Carlson GA, Kingsbury DT, Goodman PA, Coleman S, Marshall ST, DeArmond S, Westaway D, Prusiner SB (1986) Linkage of prion protein and scrapie incubation time genes. Cell 46:503–511

Carlson GA, Goodman PA, Lovett M, Taylor BA, Marshall ST, Peterson TM, Westaway D, Prusiner SB (1988) Genetics and polymorphism of the mouse prion gene complex control of scrapie incubation time. Mol Cell Biol 8:5528–5540

Carlson GA, Westaway D, DeArmond SJ, Peterson Torchia M, Prusiner SB (1989) Primary structure of prion protein may modify scrapie isolate properties. Proc Natl Acad Sci USA 86:7475–7479

Cashman NR, Loertscher R, Nalbantoglu J, Shaw I, Kascsak RJ, Bolton DC, Bendheim PE (1990) Cellular isoform of the scrapie agent protein participates in lymphocyte activation. Cell 61:185–192

Chesebro B, Race R, Wehrly K, Nishio J, Bloom M, Lechner D, Bergstrom S, Robbins K, Mayer L, Keith JM, Garon C, Haase A (1985) Identification of scrapie prion protein-specific messenger RNA in scrapie-infected and uninfected brain. Nature 315:331–333

Dickinson AG, Outram GW (1988) Genetic aspects of unconventional virus infections: the basis of the virino hypothesis. Ciba Found Symp 135:63–83

Dickinson AG, Meikle VM, Fraser H (1968) Identification of a gene which controls the incubation period of some strains of scrapie agent in mice. J Comp Pathol 78:293–299

Diedrich J, Wietgrefe S, Zupancic M et al. (1987) The molecular pathogenesis of astrogliosis in scrapie and Alzheimer's disease. Microb Pathog 2/6:435–442

Diringer H, Gelderblom H, Hilmert H, Ozel M, Edelbluth C, Kimberlin RH (1983) Scrapie infectivity, fibrils and low molecular weight protein. Nature 306:476–478

Elkins T, Zinn K, McAllister L, Hoffmann FM, Goodman CS (1990) Genetic analysis of a Drosphila neural cell adhesion molecule: interaction of fasciclin I and Abelson tyrosine kinase mutations. Cell 60:565–575

Ferguson EL, Horvitz HR (1989) The multivulva phenotype of certain Caenorhabditis elegans mutants results from defects in two functionally redundant pathways. Genetics 123:109–121

Gabizon R, McKinley MP, Groth D, Prusiner SB (1988) Immunoaffinity purification and neutralization of scrapie prion infectivity. Proc Natl Acad Sci USA 85:6617–6621

Gajdusek DC (1977) Unconventional viruses and the origin and dissappearance of Kuru. Science 197:943–960

Gibbs CJ Jr, Gajdusek DC, Asher DM, Alpers MP, Beck E, Daniel PM, Matthews WB (1968) Creutzfeld-Jakob disease (spongiform encephalopathy); Transmission to the chimpanzee. Science 161:388–389

Goebl MG, Peters TD (1986) Most of the yeast genomic sequences are not essential for cell growth and division. Cell 46:983–992

Gordon WS (1946) Vet Rec 58:516

Hämmerling GJ, Rüsch E, Tada N, Kimura S, Hämmerling U (1982) Localization of allodeterminants on H-2Kb antigens determined with monoclonal antibodies and H-2 mutant mice. Proc Natl Acad Sci USA 79:4737–4741

Hecker R, Taraboulos A, Scott M, Pan KM, Yang SL, Torchia M, Jendroska K, DeArmond SJ, Prusiner SB (1992) Replication of distinct scrapie prion isolates is region specific in brains of transgenic mice and hamsters. Genes Dev 6:1213–1228

Hooper ML, Hardy K, Handyside A, Hunter S, Monk M (1987) HPRT-deficient (Lesh-Nyhan) mouse embryos derived from germline colonization by cultured cells. Nature 326: 292–295

Hope H, Manson J (1992) The scrapie fibril protein and its cellular isoform. Curr Top Microbiol Immunol 1991: Vol 172, p 5

Hope J, Morton LJ, Farquhar CF, Multhaup G, Beyreuther K, Kimberlin RH (1986) The major polypeptide of scrapie-associated fibrils (SAF) has the same size, charge distribution and N-terminal protein sequence as predicted for the normal brain protein (PrP). EMBO J 5:2591–2597

Hsiao K, Baker HF, Crow TJ, Poulter M, Owen F, Terwilliger JD, Westaway D, Ott J, Prusiner SB (1989) Linkage of a prion protein missense variant to Gerstmann-Sträussler syndrome. Nature 338:342–345

Hsiao K, Scott M, Foster D, Groth DF, DeArmond SJ, Prusiner SB (1990) Spontaneous neurodegeneration in transgenic mice with mutant prion protein. Science 250:1587–1590

Hunter N, Hope J, McConnell I, Dickinson AG (1987) Linkage of the scrapie-associated fibril protein (PrP) gene and Sinc using congenic mice and restriction fragment length polymorphism analysis. J Gen Virol 68:2711–2716

Joyner AL, Herrup K, Auerbach BA, Davis CA, Rossant J (1991) Subtle cerebellar phenotype in mice homozygous for a targeted deletion of the En-2 homeobox. Science 251:1239–1243

Kellings K, Meyer N, Mirenda C, Prusiner SB, Riesner D (1992) Further analysis of nucleic acids in purified scrapie prion preparations by improved return refocussing gel electrophoresis. J Gen Virol 73:1025–1029

Kimberlin RH (1990) Scrapie and possible relationship with viroids. Semin Virol 1:153–162

Koch N, Hämmerling GJ, Tada N, Kimura S, Hämmerling U (1982) Cross-blocking studies with monoclonal antibodies against I-A molecules of haplotypes b, d and k. Eur J Immunol 12:909–914

Koller BH, Marrack P, Kappler JW, Smithies O (1990) Normal development of mice deficient in beta 2M, MHC class I proteins, and CD8+ T cells. Science 248:1227–1230

Latarjet R, Muel B, Haig DA, Clarke MC, Alper T (1970) Inactivation of the scrapie agent by near monochromatic ultraviolet light. Nature 227:1341–1343

Lipp HP, Van der Loos H (1991) A computer-controlled Y-maze for testing vibrosso-tactile descrimination learning in mice. Behav Brain Res 45:135–145

Manson J, Mcbride P, Hope J (1992) Expression of the PrP gene in the brain of sinc congenic mice and its relationship to the development of scrapie. Neurodegeneration 1:45–52

Masters CL, Gajdusek DC, Gibbs J Jr (1981a) Creutzfeld-Jakob disease virus isolations from the Gerstmann-Sträussler syndrome. Brain 104:559–588

Masters CL, Gajdusek DC, Gibbs CJ Jr (1981b) The familial occurence of Creutzfeld-Jakob disease and Alzheimer's disease. Brain 104:535–558

McKinley MP, Taraboulos A, Kenaga L, Serban D, DeArmond SJ, Stieber A, Prusiner SB, Gonatas N (1990) Ultrastructural localization of scrapie prion proteins in secondary lysosomes of infected cultured cells. J Cell Biol 111 (5, part 2):316a

McKinley MP, Meyer RK, Kenaga L, Rahbar F, Cotter R, Serban A, Prusiner SB (1991) Scrapie prion rod formation in vetro requires both detergent extraction and limited proteolysis. J Virol 65:1340–1351

Meyer N, Rosenbaum V, Schmidt B, Gilles K, Mirenda C, Groth D, Prusinger SB, Riesner D (1991) Search for a putative scrapie genome in purified prion fractions reveals a paucity of nucleic acids. J Gen Virol 72:37–49

Morris RGM (1984) Development of a water-maze procedure for studying spatial learning in the rat. J Neurosci Meth 11:47–60

Oesch B, Westaway D, Walchli M, McKinley MP, Kent SB, Aebersold R, Barry RA, Tempst P, Teplow DB, Hood LE et al. (1985) A cellular gene encodes scrapie PrP 27-30 protein. Cell 40:735–746

Oesch B, Groth DF, Prusiner SB, Weissmann C (1988) Search for a scrapie-specific nucleic acid: a progress report. Ciba Found Symp 135:209–223

Pattison IH (1965) Resistance of the scrapie agent to formalin. J Comp Path 74:159–164

Pattison IH (1966) The relative susceptibility of sheep, goats and mice to two types of the goat scrapie agent. Res Vet Sci 7:207–212

Prusiner SB (1982) Novel proteinaceous infectious particles cause scrapie. Science 216:136–144

Prusiner SB (1989) Scrapie prions. Annu Rev Microbiol 43:345–374

Prusiner SB (1991) Molecular biology of prion diseases. Science 252:1515–1522

Prusiner SB, DeArmond SJ (1990) Prion diseases of the central nervous system. Monogr Pathol 32:86–122

Prusiner SB, Bolton DC, Groth DF, Bowman KA, Cochran SP, McKinley MP (1982) Further purification and characterization of scrapie prions. Biochemistry 21:6942–6950

Prusiner SB, McKinley MP, Bowman KA, Bolton DC, Bendheim PE, Groth DF, Glenner GG (1983) Scrapie prions aggregate to form amyloid-like birefringent rods. Cell 35:349–358

Prusiner SB, Scott M, Foster D, Pan KM, Groth D, Mirenda C, Torchia M, Yang SL, Serban D, Carlson GA et al. (1990) Transgenetic studies implicate interactions between homologous PrP isoforms in scrapie prion replication. Cell 63:673–686

Race RE, Graham K, Ernst D, Caughey B, Chesebro B (1990) Analysis of linkage between scrapie incubation period and the prion protein gene in mice. J Gen Virol 71:493–497

Rohwer RG (1991) The scrapie agent: "a virus by any other name". Curr Top Microbiol Immunol 172:195–232

Schorle H, Holtschke T, Hunig T, Schimpl A, Horak I (1991) Development and function of T cells in mice rendered interleukin-2 deficient by gene targeting. Nature 352:621–624

Scott M, Foster D, Mirenda C, Serban D, Coufal F, Wälchli M, Torchia M, Groth D, Carlson G, DeArmond SJ, Westaway D, Prusiner SB (1989) Transgenic mice expressing hamster prion protein produce species-specific scrapie infectivity and amyloid plaques. Cell 59:847–857

Sklaviadis T, Akowitz A, Manuelidis EE, Manuelidis L (1990) Nuclease treatment results in high specific purification of Creutzfeld-Jakob disease infectivity with a density characteristic of nucleic acid-protein complexes. Arch Virol 112:215–228

Stahl N, Borchelt DR, Hsiao K, Prusiner SB (1987) Scrapie prion protein contains a phosphatidylinositol glycolipid, Cell 51:229–240

Taraboulos A, Serban D, Prusiner SB (1990) Scrapie prion proteins accumulate in the cytoplasm of persistently infected cultured cells. J Cell Biol 110:2117–2132

Turk E, Teplow DB, Hood LE, Prusiner SB (1988) Purification and properties of the cellular and scrapie hamster prion proteins. Eur J Biochem 176:21–30

Weissmann C (1991a) Spongiform encephalopathies. The prion's progress (news). Nature 349:569–571

Weissmann C (1991b) A "unified theory" of prion propagation. Nature 352:679–683

Zijlstra M, Bix M, Simister NE, Loring JM, Raulet DH, Jaenisch R (1990) Beta 2-microglobulin deficient mice lack CD4-8+ cytolytic T cells. Nature 344:742–746

4 The Carboxyterminal Fragment of the Alzheimer Amyloid Protein Precursor Causes Neurodegeneration In Vivo

Rachael L. Neve, Michael R. Kozlowski, Anja Kammerscheidt, and Christine F. Hohmann

4.1 Introduction

The neuropathology of Alzheimer's disease (AD) is characterized both by the deposition of amyloid in senile plaques and along the walls of the cerebral blood vessels (Terry et al. 1983; Glenner 1983) and also by the degeneration of neurons, which is accompanied by the intracellular formation of neurofibrillary tangles. The 39-43 amino acid fragment termed β/A4 (Glenner and Wong 1984a,b; Masters et al. 1985) is the primary component of the amyloid deposits. The isolation of complementary DNAs (cDNAs) containing the β/A4 coding sequence by our laboratory and others (Tanzi et al. 1987; Kang et al. 1987; Goldgaber et al. 1987; Robakis et al. 1987) revealed that the β/A4 found in amyloid deposits in AD represents a peptide derived from a larger precursor protein.

The mechanism of β/A4 production in AD remains unclear. Its parent molecule, βAPP, is a transmembrane protein in which the β/A4 peptide spans the border between the extracellular domain and the transmembrane region (Kang et al. 1987; Weidemann et al. 1989; Selkoe et al. 1988). Normal cleavage of APP occurs predominantly at LYS_{16} (Sisodia et al. 1990; Esch et al. 1990; Anderson et al. 1991), thereby releasing protease nexin-II (Van Nostrand et al. 1989; Oltersdorf et al. 1989). In addition, a minor lysosomal processing pathway in the brain appears to yield several potentially amyloidogenic β/A4-containing carboxyterminal fragments with heterogeneous aminotermini (Golde et al. 1992; Estus et al. 1992). Thus, the pathological accumulation of the β/A4 polypeptide in AD brain does not necessarily result from an abnormal cleavage event, but may instead accrue from a cellular shift to the lysosomal processing pathway for βAPP or from inappropriate post-translational modification of a normal carboxyterminal processing product.

Because the carboxyterminus of β/A4 is within the transmembrane domain of βAPP, where it is not normally accessible to proteases, its cleavage may be a secondary event (Spillantini et al. 1990). Thus, we initially sought to determine not only whether β/A4 itself is neurotoxic, but also whether the carboxyterminal 100 amino acids of βAPP (which would presumably be the initial product of a cleavage of βAPP at the amino terminus of the β/A4 sequence) can cause neurodegeneration. Recent evidence from our laboratory and others has indeed implicated the 100 amino acid carboxyterminal fragment of βAPP in the processes of both amyloidogenesis and neurodegeneration. This fragment, which spans the β/A4 and cytoplasmic domains, has a tendency to self-aggregate (Dyrks et al. 1988). Moreover, the expression of this carboxyterminal βAPP fragment in primate cells has been shown to lead to the production of a 16-kDa protein which aggregates and accumulates into deposit-like structures (Wolf et al. 1990), and that results in the formation of amyloid-like fibrils (Maruyama et al. 1990).

We have shown that this same carboxyterminal APP fragment is neurotoxic (Yankner et al. 1989). The neurotoxicity of this carboxyterminal βAPP fragment suggests that it may play a role not only in amyloidogenesis but also in the development of the progressive neuropathology of AD. We present below pharmacological evidence suggesting that the neurotoxicity of βAPP-C100 is mediated by its specific binding to a neuronal cell surface molecule. We also describe two animal models that we have developed to analyze the neurodegenerative properties of βAPP-C100.

4.2 βAPP-C100 Is Toxic Specifically to Neurons

PC12 cells transfected with a retroviral recombinant expressing the carboxyterminal 100 amino acids of βAPP (formerly termed AB1, Yankner et al. 1989; and then βAPP-C104, Kozlowski et al. 1992; now termed βAPP-C100) degenerate when induced to differentiate into neuronal cells with nerve growth factor (NGF; Yankner et al. 1989). Moreover, conditioned medium from these cells, but not from control cells transfected with recombinant βAPP-695 or from cells transfected with recombinants expessing β/A4, is toxic to neurons but not non-neuronal cells in primary rat hippocampal cultures (Fig. 1). As shown

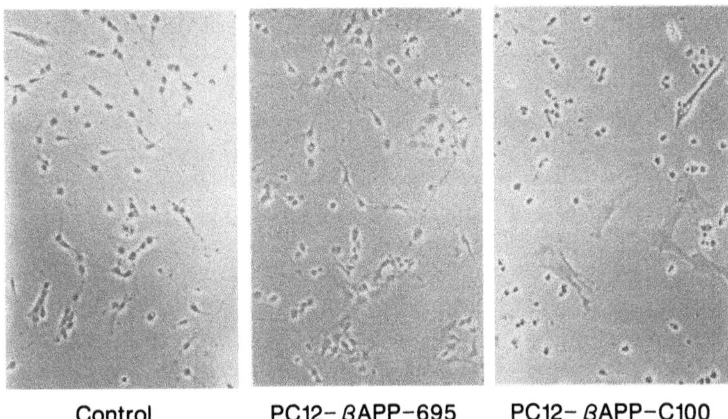

Fig. 1. Appearance of primary rat hippocampal cultures 4 days after plating, in the presence of mock-conditioned medium (control), conditioned medium from control βAPP-695 transfected PC12 cells, and conditioned medium from βAPP-C100 transfected PC12 cells. Note extensive neuronal death (but sparing of glia) only in the cultures treated with βAPP-C100 conditioned medium

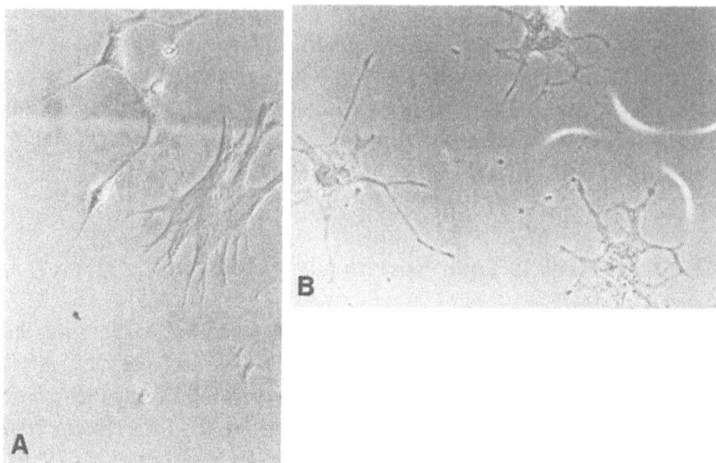

Fig. 2A,B. Glial cells are spared following treatment of primary rat hippocampal cultures with βAPP-C100 conditioned medium. Note also that neurons adjacent to glial cells (see, for example **A**) are often protected from the toxicity

in Figs. 1 and 2, βAPP-C100 has deleterious effects on neurons but not on glia in primary cultures. Moreover, neurons adjacent to glial cells (Fig. 2A) are often protected from the toxicity. Addition of βAPP-C100 conditioned medium to primary hippocampal cultures reveals a specific pattern of degeneration of the neurons (Fig. 3). Neuronal processes are retracted, leading to the appearance of stunted processes (Fig. 3B), which in some cases display abnormal branching. Extensive fasciculation of nonretracted processes (Fig. 3C) is often accompanied by severe clumping of the neurons (Fig. 3D). The neurotoxicity can be removed from the medium by immunoabsorption with an antibody to βAPP-C100 (Yankner et al. 1989), suggesting that βAPP-C100 is secreted by the transfected cells and is neurotoxic.

We extended our characterization of the mechanism by which βAPP-C100 may kill neurons by evaluating the pH dependence of the toxicity and by assessing the functional effects of site-directed in vitro mutagenesis of βAPP-C100 (Kozlowski et al. 1992). Because we had noted that differentiated PC12 cells were relatively resistant to βAPP-C100 toxicity under alkaline conditions, we first examined βAPP-

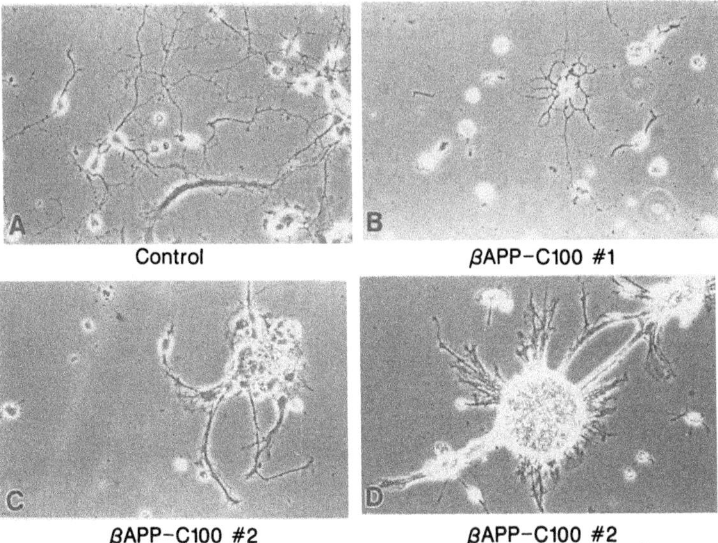

Fig. 3A–D. Appearance of surviving neurons in rat hippocampal cultures treated with βAPP-C100 conditioned medium for 4 days

C100 neurotoxicity in medium at pH 7.3, compared with that in medium at pH 8.0 (Fig. 4). We discovered that βAPP-C100 transfectants displayed no detectable degeneration at pH 8.0 even after 9 days of treatment with NGF, whereas neurodegeneration of the transfectants was apparent by day 6 of NGF treatment at pH 7.3. We then exposed control and experimental transfected PC12 cell lines to NGF in media at pH ranging from pH 7.2 (medium at pH lower than 7.2 was slightly toxic to control cells) to pH 8.2 in 0.1 pH unit increments. The data revealed that the neurotoxicity of βAPP-C100 is dependent upon pH and is almost completely inhibited at pH 7.8 or above.

The aminoterminal sequence of βAPP-C100 contains a tyrosine (687 in βAPP-695) that lies within a sequence homologous to the sequence surrounding a phosphorylated tyrosine in integrins and some plasma membrane receptors (reviewed by Tamkun et al. 1986). This homology suggested that tyrosine 687 in βAPP-C100 might be important to its function. We used site-directed mutagenesis to replace the ty-

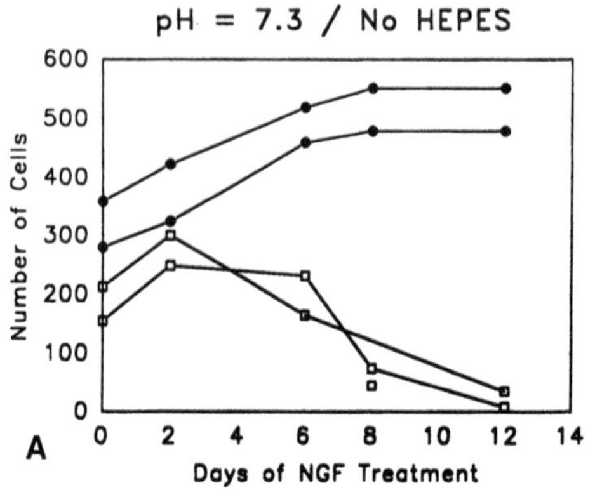
pH = 7.3 / No HEPES
Number of Cells
600
500
400
300
200
100
0
0 2 4 6 8 10 12 14
Days of NGF Treatment
A

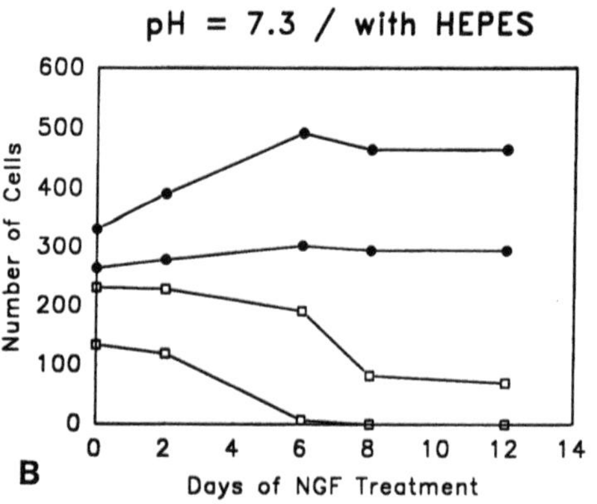
pH = 7.3 / with HEPES
Number of Cells
600
500
400
300
200
100
0
0 2 4 6 8 10 12 14
Days of NGF Treatment
B

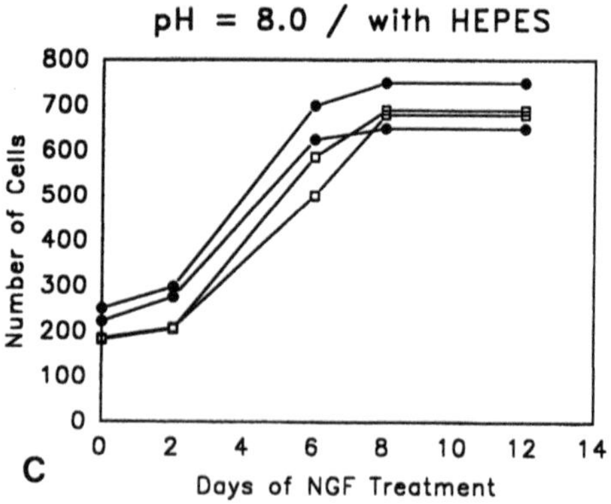
pH = 8.0 / with HEPES
Number of Cells
800
700
600
500
400
300
200
100
0
0 2 4 6 8 10 12 14
Days of NGF Treatment
C

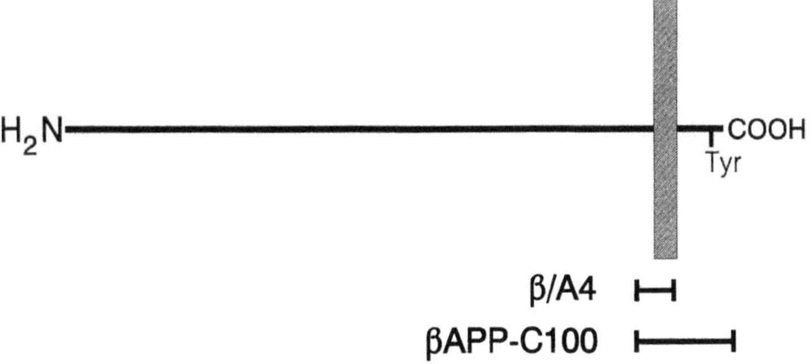

Characteristics of βAPP-C100 Toxicity

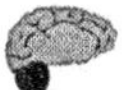
Specific for neuronal cells (protection by glia)

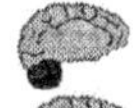
Dependent upon pH

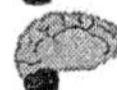
Abolished by removal of Tyr 687

Fig. 5. Schematic drawing showing positions of β/A4 and βAPP-C100 within the βAPP coding sequence; a summary of the characteristics of βAPP-C100 toxicity are presented in the *lower half of the panel*. These characteristics should be compared with those of βAPP-C100 binding, detailed in Fig. 6

rosine with a phenylalanine. Conditioned medium from the mutant transfectants was not toxic to NGF-treated cells (Kozlowski et al. 1992), suggesting that tyrosine 687 is necessary for the neurotoxicity of βAPP-C100, either as a site for phosphorylation or as an internalization sequence. The characteristics of βAPP-C100 toxicity are summarized in Fig. 5.

Fig. 4A–C. pH dependence of βAPP-C100 neurotoxicity. The growth of control vector-transfected PC12 cells (DO-PC12, *filled circles*) is largely unaffected by changes in pH, whereas βAPP-C100 (*open squares*) expressing transfectants gradually die at pH 7.3 but not at pH 8.0

4.3 The Neurotoxicity of βAPP-C100 May Be Mediated by Its Binding to a Neuronal Cell Surface Molecule

We synthesized ^{35}S-labeled βAPP-C100 in vitro and showed that it binds to a site on the surface of NGF-treated PC12 cells that has several receptor-like properties (Kozlowski et al. 1992). First, this cell surface molecule binds βAPP-C100, as demonstrated in dissociation experiments. Second, the binding of ^{35}S-labeled β-A0PP-C100 to the cell surface molecule is specific: binding is inhibited by unlabeled βAPP-C100 (Fig. 6) but not inhibited by other peptides, including tachykinins. Third, βAPP-C100 is not altered after binding as shown by SDS-PAGE analysis of the ligand. Finally, the binding site has high (nanomolar) affinity and low capacity, as would be expected for a receptor.

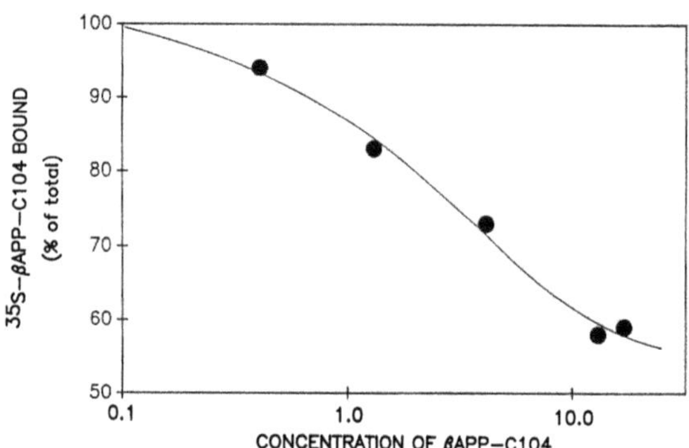

Characteristics of βAPP-C100 Binding

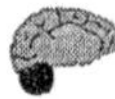 Specific for neuronal cells

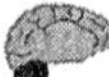 Dependent upon pH

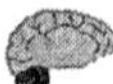 Abolished by removal of Tyr 687

Fig. 6. Summary of characteristics of βAPP-C100 binding to a neuronal cell surface receptor, underneath a representative curve showing the inhibition of ^{35}S-labeled βAPP-C100 binding to NGF-treated (5 days) PC12 cells by βAPP-C100

Three of our results (Fig. 6) provide circumstantial evidence that this binding site mediates the toxic effects of βAPP-C100 on differentiated PC12 cells. First, the binding site is much more prevalent on PC12 cells rendered susceptible to the toxic effects of βAPP-C100 by treatment with NGF than on nontreated cells, to which the peptide is not toxic (Yankner et al. 1989). Second, a loss of both binding and toxicity occurs near pH 7.8. Third, a mutation that eliminates the neurotoxic efficacy of βAPP-C100 (tyrosine 687) also abolishes its ability to bind to the site identified in this study.

4.4 Transplantation of Transfected PC12 Cells into Brains of Mice – Results in Neuropathology

PC12 cells transfected with the βAPP-C100 retroviral recombinant, or with the retroviral vector alone, were transplanted into the hippocampocortical region of postnatal day (PD) 1-2 or PD6 mice (Fig. 7; this work is described in Neve et al. 1992). Clusters of grafted PC12 cells were clearly evident in both the experimental (βAPP-C100) and con-

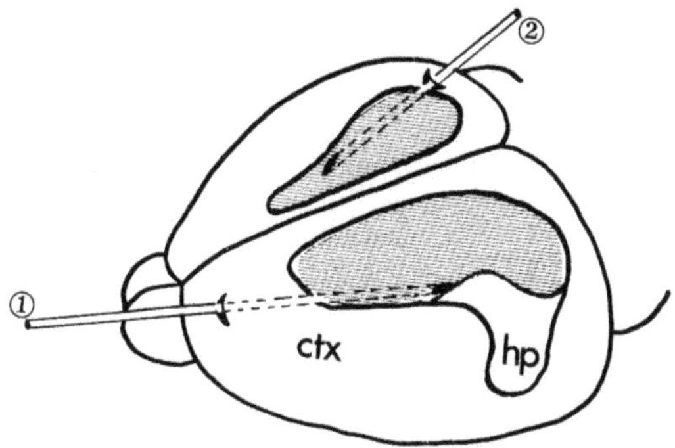

Fig. 7. Diagrammatic representation of the transplant procedure. A bevelled glass capillary containing cell suspension was inserted through skin and skull of anesthetized pups into the brain parenchema and run towards the dorsal hippocampo-cortical area in parallel to the brain surface. Cell suspension was injected near the indicated tip of the capillary. The two different placement strategies employed are indicated by *1*, antero-to-posterior, and *2*, postero-to-anterior. Both approaches yielded similar results. *ctx*, cortex; *hp*, hippocampus

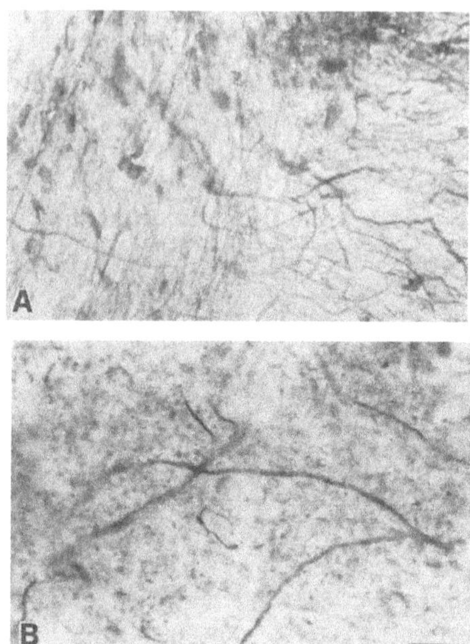

Fig. 8 A,B. Alz-50 immunoreactivity in a 4-month-old animal transplanted with βAPP-C100 transfected PC12 cells (**A**) and in AD brain (**B**). **A** Alz-50 immunoreactivity in the cortex adjacent to the neurodegeneration in 4-month-old post-transplant animals reveals abnormal dystrophic-appearing fibers similar in appearance to those immunoreactive with Alz-50 in the temporal cortex of an individual with histopathologically diagnosed Alzheimer's disease. *Scale bar* is 25 μm

trol animals (DO vector only) sacrificed 20 days following transplantation), although these clusters had largely disappeared by 2 months after transplantation, leaving only scars to mark the locations of the transplants. At 4 months after transplantation, experimental animals exhibited significant cortical atrophy relative to controls; this atrophy was not evident at the earlier age of 2 months. Some of the mice that had been transplanted with βAPP-C100 transfected cells also revealed immunoreactivity with Alz-50, an antibody that detects an AD related protein (Wolozin et al. 1986), in the somatodendritic domain of neurons in the cortex surrounding the transplants, and in dystrophic-appearing fibers in the same region (Fig. 8). In addition, abnormal organization of the neuropil in the CA2/3 region of the hippocampus ipsilateral to the transplant was revealed by immunostaining with F5, an antibody to the carboxyterminal end of the amyloid protein precursor. Adjacent Nissl-stained sections did not reveal gross morphological abnormalities in the area of decreased F5 staining, suggesting that the disorganization evident in the immunostained section mainly involves neuropil at 4 months after transplantation. Together, these results suggest that the carboxyterminal fragment of βAPP may cause specific neuropathology and neurodegeneration in vivo.

4.5 Transgenic Mice Expressing βAPP-C100 in the Brain Display AD-like Neuropathology

The neuropathological effects resulting from transplantation of βAPP-C100 transfected cells into the mouse brain suggests that it may play a role not only in amyloidogenesis but also in the neurodegeneration of AD. To test further this hypothesis, we expressed βAPP-C100 in the brains of transgenic mice under the control of the dystrophin brain promoter (Kammesheidt et al., in press). These mice display, at 4 months of age, intraneuronal deposition of the β/A4 protein, abnormal intracellular accumulations of a carboxyterminal epitope of βAPP that is similar to that we previously described in AD brain (Fig. 9; Benowitz et al. 1989), and thioflavin S fluorescence around blood vessels in the brain (Fig. 10).

Electrophysiological analysis of hippocampal slices from 1-year-old transgenic mice and control sibs suggests severe loss of functional synapses in the transgenic mice relative to controls and to 2-month-old transgenic mice. The loss of synaptic function, revealed as potentials less robust than those of controls, is more apparent in the CA1 region of the hippocampus than in the dentate (R. Malenka, personal communication). This pattern of functional synaptic loss is similar to the pattern of neurodegeneration in the AD hippocampus. Thus, these mice may be a useful model for describing the progression of events that culminates in the manifestation of specific aspects of AD pathology and ultimately for developing a strategy to halt this progression.

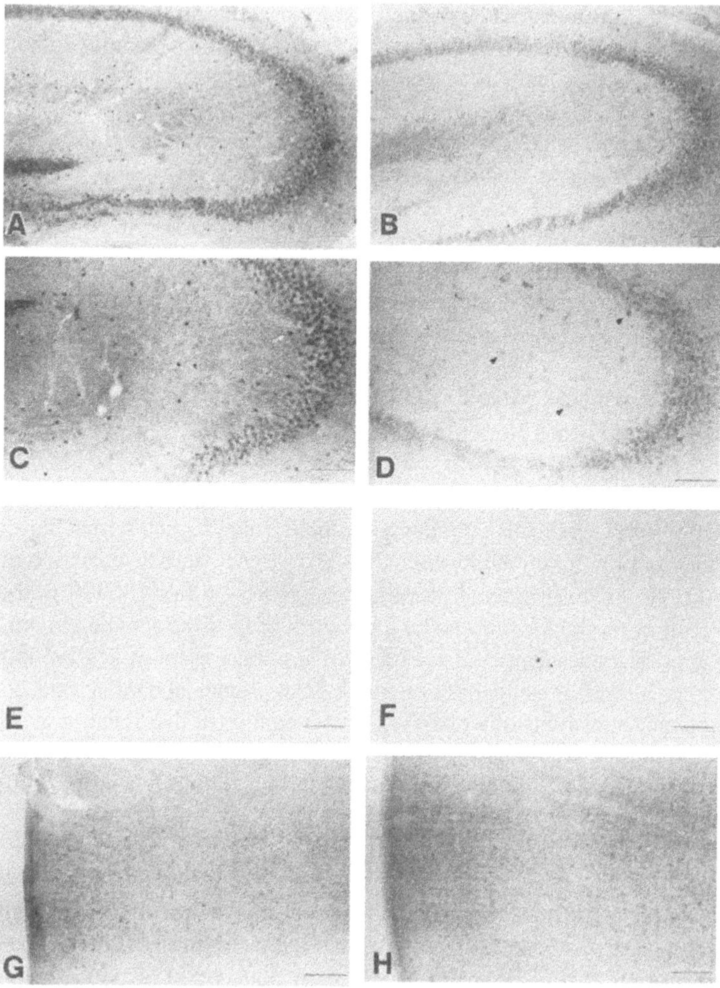

Fig. 9A–H. E1-42 immunoreactivity in the hippocampus of a transgenic animal (**A** and **C** are different magnifications) compared with that of a control animal (**B,D**). While low-level staining of cell bodies in the pyramidal cell layer and in additional scattered cells is seen in the control mouse (**D**, *arrowheads*), darker punctate accumulations of E1-42 immunoreactivity in the pyramidal cell layer and throughout the hippocampus (**C**, *arrows*) are unique to the transgenic mice. Preabsorption of the E1-42 antibody with 30 μg of pep-

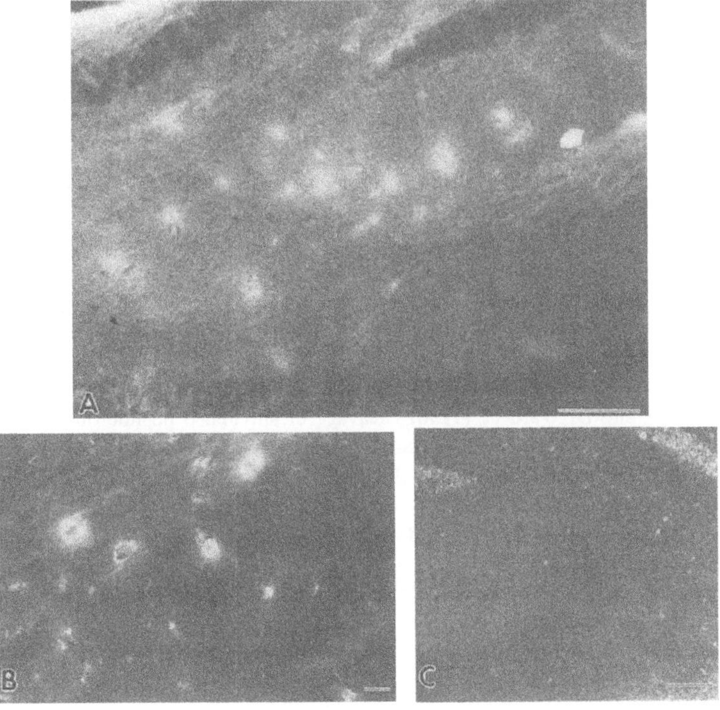

Fig. 10A–C. Thioflavin S fluorescence around blood vessels in the hippo-campus of a transgenic mouse from line 2. **A,B** Different magnifications of the fluorescence. No abnormal thioflavin S fluorescence was visible in control mice (**C**). Note that the image shown in (**C**) was the result of an exposure time five times that of the images shown in **A** and **B**. The light fluorescence of the pyramidal cell layer was evident in all animals, including controls; it does not show up in **A** and **B** because the perivascular fluorescence is so much brighter that it effectively quenches the pyramidal cell layer fluorescence. The *scale bar* in **A** and **C** represents 100 μm; the *bar* in **B** represents 10 μm

tide/μl of antibody results in absence of staining as shown in **E** (transgenic mouse) and **F** (control mouse). **G,H** E1-42 immunoreactivity in the parietal cortex of a transgenic mouse (**G**) and a control mouse (**H**). Differences in E1-42 immunoreactivity between transgenic and control mice in the parietal cortex are much less pronounced than in the hippocampus. All comparisons of transgenic and control mice were made using tissue processed in parallel and developed with DAB for equivalent periods of time. The *scale bars* represent 100 μm

References

Anderson JP, Esch FS, Keim PS, Sambamurti K, Lieberburg I, Robakis NK (1991) Exact cleavage site of Alzheimer amyloid precursor in neuronal PC-12 cells. Neurosci Letters 128:126-128

Benowitz LI, Rodriguez W, Paskevich P, Mufson EJ, Schenk D, Neve RL (1989) The amyloid precursor protein is concentrated in neuronal lysosomes in normal and Alzheimer disease subjects. Exp Neurol 106:237-250

Dyrks T, Weidemann A, Multhaup G, Salbaum JM, Lemaire HG, Kang J, Müller-Hill B, Masters CL, Beyreuther K (1988) Identification, transmembrane orientation and biogenesis of the amyloid A4 precursor of Alzheimer's disease. EMBO J 7:49-957

Esch FS, Keim PS, Beattie EC, Blacher RW, Culwell AR, Oltersdorf T, McClure D, Ward PJ (1990) Cleavage of amyloid β peptide during constitutive processing of its precursor. Science 248:1122-1124

Estus S, Golde TE, Kunishita T, Blades D, Lowery D, Eisen M, Usiak M, Qu, Xuemei, Tabira T, Greenberg GD, Younkin SG (1992) Potentially amyloidogenic, carboxyl-terminal derivatives of the amyloid protein precursor. Science 255: 726-728

Glenner GG (1983) Alzheimer's disease: The commonest form of amyloidosis. Arch Pathol Lab Med 107:281-282

Glenner GG, Wong CW (1984a) Alzheimer's disease: initial report of the purification and characterization of a novel cerebrovascular amyloid protein. Biochem Biophys Res Commun 120:885-890

Glenner GG, Wong CW (1984b) Alzheimer's disease and Down's syndrome: sharing of a unique cerebrovascular amyloid protein. Biochem Biophys Res Commun 122:1131-1135

Golde TE, Estus S, Younkin LH, Selkoe DJ, Younkin SG (1992) Processing of the amyloid protein precursor to potentially amyloidogenic derivatives. Science 255:728-730

Goldgaber D, Lerman MI, McBride W, Saffiotti U, Gajdusek DC (1987) Characterization and chromosomal localization of a cDNA encoding brain amyloid of Alzheimer's disease. Science 235:877-880

Kammesheidt A, Boyce FM, Spanoyannis AF, Cummings BJ, Ortegon M, Cotman CW, Vaught JL, Neve RL. Deposition of β/A4 immunoreactivity and neuronal pathology in transgenic mice expressing the carboxyterminal fragment of the Alzheimer amyloid precursor in the brain. Proc Natl Acad Sci USA, in press

Kang J, Lemaire HG, Unterbeck A, Salbaum MJ, Masters CL, Grzeschik KH, Multhaup G, Beyreuther K, and Muller-Hill B (1987) The precursor of

Alzheimer's disease amyloid A4 protein resembles a cell surface receptor. Nature 325:733-736

Kozlowski MR, Spanoyannis A, Manly SP, Fidel SA, Neve RL (1992) The neurotoxic carboxyterminal fragment of the Alzheimer amyloid precursor binds specifically to a neuronal cell surface molecule: pH dependence of the neurotoxicity and the binding. J Neurosci 12:1679-1687

Maruyama K, Terakado K, Usami M, Yoshikawa K (1990) Formation of amyloid-like fibrils in COS cells overexpressing part of the Alzheimer amyloid protein precursor. Nature 347:566-569

Masters CL, Simms G, Weinman NA, Multhaup G, McDonald BL, Beyreuther K. (1985) Amyloid plaque core protein in Alzheimer disease and Down syndrome. Proc Natl Acad Sci USA 82:4245-4249

Neve RL, Kammesheidt A, Hohmann CF (1992) Brain transplants of cells expressing the carboxyterminal fragment of the Alzheimer amyloid precursor cause specific neuropathology *in vivo*. Proc Natl Acad Sci USA 89:3448-3452

Oltersdorf T, Fritz LC, Schenk DB, Lieberburg I, Johnson-Wood KL, Beattie EC, Ward PJ, Blacher RW, Dovey HF, Sinha S (1989) The secreted form of the Alzheimer's amyloid precursor protein with the Kunitz domain is protease nexin-II. Nature 341:144-147

Robakis NK, Ramakrishna N, Wolfe G, Wisniewski HM (1987) Molecular cloning and characterization of a cDNA encoding the cerebrovascular and the neurite plaque amyloid peptides. Proc Natl Acad Sci USA 84:4190-4194

Selkoe DJ, Podlisny MB, Joachim CL, Vickers EA, Lee G, Fritz LC, Oltersdorf T (1988) β-amyloid precursor protein of Alzheimer disease occurs as 110-135-kilodalton membrane-associated proteins in neural and non-neural tissues. Proc Natl Acad Sci USA 85:7341-7345

Sisodia SS, Koo EH, Beyreuther K, Unterbeck A, Price DL (1990) Evidence that β-amyloid protein in Alzheimer's disease is not derived by normal processing. Science 248:492-495

Spillantini MG, Goedert M, Jakes R, Klug A (1990) Different configurational states of β-amyloid and their distributions relative to plaques and tangles in Alzheimer disease. Proc Natl Acad Sci USA 87:3947-3951

Tamkun JW, DeSimone DW, Fonda D, Patel RS, Buck C, Horwitz AF, Hynes RO (1986) Structure of integrin, a glycoprotein involved in the transmembrane linkage between fibronectin and actin. Cell 46:271-282

Tanzi RE, Gusella JF, Watkins PC, Bruns GAP, St. George-Hyslop P, Van Keuren M, Patterson D, Pagan S, Kurnit DM, Neve RL (1987) Amyloid β-protein gene: cDNA, mRNA distribution, and genetic linkage near the Alzheimer locus. Science 235:880-884

Terry RD, Peck A, DeTeresa R, Schechter R, Horoupian DS (1983) Some morphometric aspects of the brain in senile dementia of the Alzheimer type. Ann Neurol 10:184-192

Van Nostrand WE, Wagner SL, Suzuki M, Choi BH, Farrow JS, Geddes JW, Cotman CW, Cunningham DD (1989) Protease nexin-II, a potent anti-chymotrypsin, shows identity to amyloid β-protein precursor. Nature 341:546-549

Weidemann A, Konig G, Bunke D, Fischer P, Salbaum JM, Masters CL, Beyreuther K (1989) Identification, biogenesis, and localization of precursors of Alzheimer's disease A4 amyloid protein. Cell 57:115-126

Wolf D, Quon D, Wang Y, Cordell B (1990) Identification and characterization of C-terminal fragments of the β-amyloid precursor produced in cell culture. EMBO J 9:2079-2084

Wolozin BL, Pruchnicki A, Dickson DW, Davies P (1986) A neuronal antigen in the brains of Alzheimer patients. Science 232:648-650

Yankner BA, Dawes LR, Fisher S, Villa-Komaroff L, Oster-Granite ML, Neve RL (1989) Neurotoxicity of a fragment of the amyloid precursor associated with Alzheimer's disease. Science 245:417-420

5 Transgenic Models of Chronic Arthritis and of Systemic Tumour Necrosis Factor-Mediated Disease in Mice Expressing Human Tumour Necrosis Factor

George A. Kollias

5.1 Introduction

Tumour necrosis factor (TNF-α/cachectin, TNF) was discovered originally as a factor displaying cytotoxic/cytostatic effects on transformed cells in vitro and necrotizing activity on certain transplantable tumours in vivo (Carswell et al. 1975). In later studies, TNF was shown to be the primary mediator of wasting accompanying chronic invasive diseases (Beutler et al. 1985; Tracey et al. 1986). Acting in concert with other members of the cytokine network, TNF has now been clearly established as a central regulator of inflammation and immunity, mainly

Table 1. In vivo activities of TNF — context, rate and duration of TNF synthesis

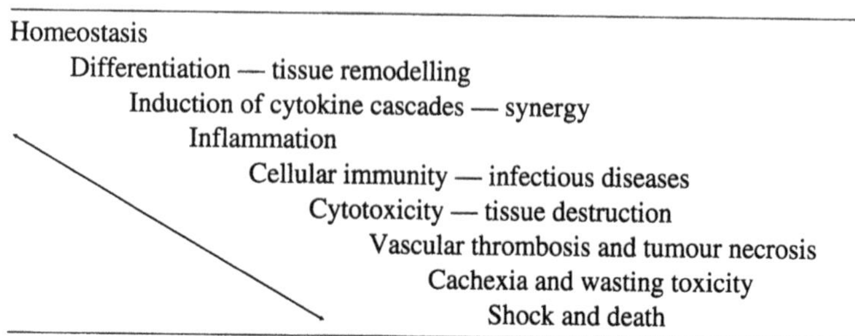

Homeostasis
Differentiation — tissue remodelling
Induction of cytokine cascades — synergy
Inflammation
Cellular immunity — infectious diseases
Cytotoxicity — tissue destruction
Vascular thrombosis and tumour necrosis
Cachexia and wasting toxicity
Shock and death

by modulating the functional state of cells that participate in such processes (reviewed by Beutler and Cerami 1989; Old 1990). For example, it has been shown that TNF augments the cytotoxicity of macrophages (Esparza et al. 1987), induces neutrophil adhesion and activation (Gamble et al. 1985) and regulates T and B cell growth and differentiation (Shalaby et al. 1988). The cell-specific effects of TNF are also exerted in a number of nonimmune cell types. The hemostatic properties of vascular endothelial cells are found to be modulated by TNF which induces the production of procoagulant activity (Nawroth and Stern 1986) and enhances the expression of adhesion molecules that bind neutrophils and monocytes (Gamble et al. 1985). Moreover, TNF is shown to be a growth factor for normal fibroblasts (Vilcek et al. 1986) and thymocytes (Ranges et al. 1988) and to interfere with the metabolism of adipocytes (Semb et al. 1987). In response to TNF many cell types are found to increase the production of several other factors, including IL-6, IL-1, colony stimulating factors, collagenase, PGE_2, c-*fos*, c-*myc* and histocompatibility antigens. Fine tuning of such circuits is very important to the defence of the host and to the restoration of homeostasis in the body following a microbial infection or a tissue injury.

Depending on the presence of other signalling molecules, the rate of production and the duration of exposure, TNF action can be either beneficial or deleterious to the host, ranging from tissue remodelling and inflammation to severe wasting and shock (Table 1). Deregulated production of TNF in humans is thought to contribute to the pathogenesis of apparently disparate disease states, such as septic shock (Beutler et al. 1985; Tracey et al. 1986), cancer-associated cachexia (Oliff et al. 1987), autoimmunity (Held et al. 1990), graft-versus-host disease (Piguet et al. 1987), cerebral malaria (Grau et al. 1989), AIDS (Osborn et al. 1989) and arthritis (Saxne et al. 1988; Yocum et al. 1989; Keffer et al. 1991).

In this chapter we shall review the current understanding of the molecular mechanisms regulating TNF gene expression and function and discuss the development of specific TNF-mediated disease in transgenic mouse lines engineered to constitutively express human TNF protein in their tissues. Transgenic systems developing arthritis, hair growth defects, localized cytotoxicity, ischaemic organ necrosis and wasting are expected to facilitate further in vivo molecular characterization of the role of TNF in triggering disease and to serve as valuable tools for optimizing preventive or therapeutic protocols aimed at treatment of related disorders in humans.

5.2 Regulation of TNF Biosynthesis and Signalling

Activated macrophages and T lymphocytes are both major cellular sources of TNF. Its production is regulated mainly at the post-transcriptional level (Beutler et al. 1986; Han et al. 1990). Thus, in resting macrophages, low levels of TNF mRNA can be detected while no protein is synthesized. Following activation by lipopolysaccharide (LPS), a major inducer of inflammation, transcription from the TNF gene is augmented 3-fold while steady-state mRNA levels are increased by 50-fold or more. In addition, a set of highly conserved UA-rich sequences located at the 3'-untranslated (3'-UTR) region of mRNAs coding for several inflammatory mediators including TNF (Caput et al. 1986) is thought to be critical in the regulation of both mRNA stability (Shaw and Kamen 1986) and translational efficiency (Kruys et al. 1989; Han et al. 1990).

Expression analysis has shown that TNF is produced both as a 17-kDa secreted form and as a 26-kDa membrane-associated form. Both molecular forms of TNF are produced by monocytic cells (Kriegler et al. 1988; Luettig et al. 1989) and T lymphocytes (Kinkhabwala et al. 1990). Membrane-associated TNF is thought to be a precursor to soluble TNF (Jue et al. 1990) and it shares cytotoxic properties towards TNF-sensitive targets (Kriegler et al. 1988). These observations have led to the hypothesis that the different molecular forms of TNF mediate different physiological effects, systemic toxicity being mediated by the deregulated production of soluble 17-kDa TNF while membrane-associated TNF might act locally in a directed, paracrine and/or contact-dependent manner.

Additional mechanisms modulate TNF activity. TNF signal transduction occurs via two distinct high-affinity receptors, the p55- (TNF-RI) and the p75-kDa (TNF-RII) TNF receptors, which are present on the surface of most cells (Smith and Baglioni 1989; Brockhaus et al. 1990). The two receptors are differentially regulated and mediate distinct cellular responses (Tartaglia et al. 1991). The murine p75-TNF-R has been found to induce signals for the proliferation of thymocytes and cytotoxic T cells, whereas the p55-TNF-R initiates signals for cytotoxicity (Tartaglia et al. 1991). The existence of both receptors also as soluble forms imposes a further regulatory mechanism on TNF action since these soluble receptors compete for TNF and thereby may function as inhibitors of TNF activity (Seckinger et al. 1989; Engelmann et al. 1989). The soluble receptors are derived from their cell surface counterparts in a regulated manner (Porteu and Nathan 1990; Kohno et al. 1990). Of relevance to our transgenic studies is the finding that the murine p75-TNF-R shows strong species specificity for murine TNF and therefore might fail to mediate signals from human TNF (Lewis et al. 1991).

It is therefore apparent that regulation of TNF action operates at multiple levels and little is known about how the different mechanisms interact in vivo to control TNF production and function. To simulate part of this biology in an in vivo experimental system, and to define the biological potential of deregulated human TNF production, we studied several transgenic mouse lines carrying and expressing wild-type or modified human TNF gene constructs.

5.3 Generation of Transgenic Mice

We have employed three types of DNA constructs as shown in Fig. 1. First, a wild-type human TNF transgene (RI-TNF gene construct) was

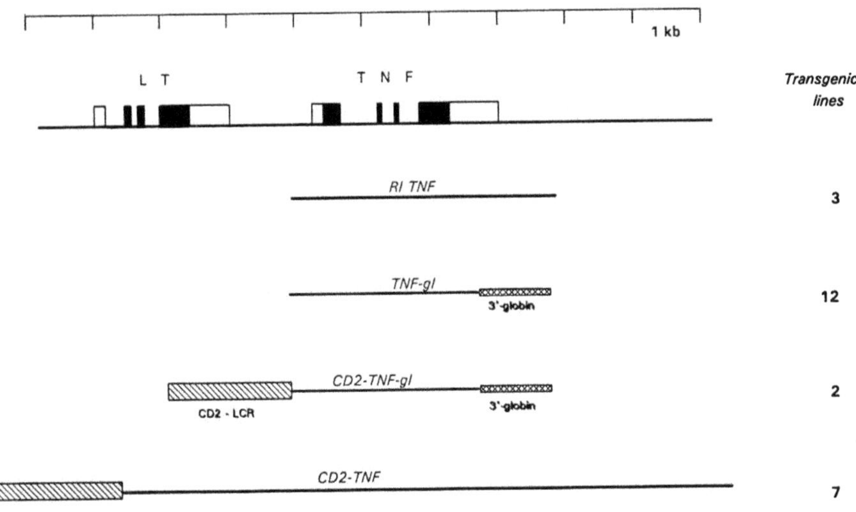

Fig. 1. Structure of human tumour necrosis factor (*TNF*) gene constructs microinjected into (CBAxC57BL/6) F_2 hybrid mouse zygotes. Map is in scale except for the CD2 genomic fragment which is 5 kb in length. *Boxes* denote exons, *filled boxes* coding sequences and *open boxes* 5' or 3' untranslated sequences. *LT*, lymphotoxin

used in order to identify the minimum DNA sequences that would be sufficient to confer correct, regulated expression of huTNF in transgenic tissues. Second, in order to overexpress TNF in transgenic tissues, we exchanged the 3'-UTR of the hutnf gene with the 3'-region of the human β-globin gene (TNF-gl gene construct; Fig. 1). This modification was suggested to us by previous findings which demonstrated that the 3'-UTR's of most cytokine mRNAS, including TNF, impose post-transcriptional regulatory constraints on their expression (Kruys et al. 1989; Han et al. 1990). Finally, to examine the biological potential of high-level, T cell-targeted expression of huTNF in transgenic mice, we designed a third type of gene construct in which wild-type or 3'-modified genomic fragments of the human TNF genetic locus were coupled to the locus control region of the gene encoding human CD2 (CD2-TNF-gl and CD2-TNF gene constructs; Fig. 1). These CD2 gene sequences have been shown to direct high-level, posi-

tion-independent and T cell-specific expression of linked heterologous
genes in transgenic mice (Greaves et al. 1989).

5.4 Patterns of huTNF Gene Expression in Transgenic Mice

Transgenic tissues were analysed for exogenous TNF mRNA expression by 5'- and 3'-specific S1 nuclease protection assays. Constitutive, low-level steady-state mRNA specific for human TNF was
detected in the thymus, lung, spleen, kidney and joints of transgenic
mice expressing both wild-type and 3'-modified TNF gene constructs.
To examine whether expression of the TNF transgenes can be regulated by LPS, peritoneal macrophages from transgenic mice were assessed for expression of mRNA, before or after induction by LPS. In
contrast to the inducible expression of the wild-type TNF gene construct, no exogenous mRNA signal could be detected in macrophages
from one of the lines constitutively expressing the 3'-modified TNF
transgene. Taken together, our results (Keffer et al. 1991) show that
correct, endotoxin responsive expression of human TNF transgenes
can be established in transgenic mice and that the necessary *cis*-acting
DNA information for this, is contained within a 3.6-kb DNA fragment.
They also suggest that the 3'-region of the human TNF gene, which is
deleted in the 3'-modified TNF-globin transgene, contains information
necessary for macrophage-specific TNF gene expression.

For the third type of construct, the CD2-LCR driven TNF transgenes, T cell-specific expression was confirmed by both RNA and protein detection assays performed in transgenic tissues. In general, high
levels of human TNF mRNA were detected in the thymus and mesenteric lymph nodes from these mice. In contrast, expression in spleen
was found to be present at much lower levels, while expression in
liver, kidney, brain, lung and gut was undetectable. Expression of
huTNF mRNA was undetectable in peritoneal macrophages from these
mice either before or after induction by LPS. Immunocytochemical
analysis performed in one of the CD2-TNF-globin transgenic lines
showed immunoreactive huTNF protein in thymic lymphocytes distributed throughout the transgenic thymus. These TNF-immunoreac-
tive lymphocytes showed both cytoplasmic and plasma membrane
staining. Immunoprecipitation experiments further showed that both

membrane-bound (26-kDa) and secreted (17-kDa) forms of TNF are produced by thymocytes of this line.

5.5 Human TNF Transgenic Mice Develop a Hair Growth Defect

A common feature of the macroscopic appearance of several huTNF transgenic mouse lines, irrespective of the type of the expressed transgene, was the development of a hair growth defect (Fig. 2) which could not be associated with histological abnormalities of skin tissue at the light-microscope level. Poor hair growth could be suppressed from birth, or neutralized at later stages, by treatment with antibodies against human TNF (kindly provided by Celltech, UK) showing that exogenous TNF acts as a specific trigger for the development of this defect, which did not appear to affect normal development. Transgenic mice showing this phenotype and no other abnormality (see below) appeared healthy and fertile. Histological examination of mice carrying the wild-type huTNF transgene did not reveal further abnormalities.

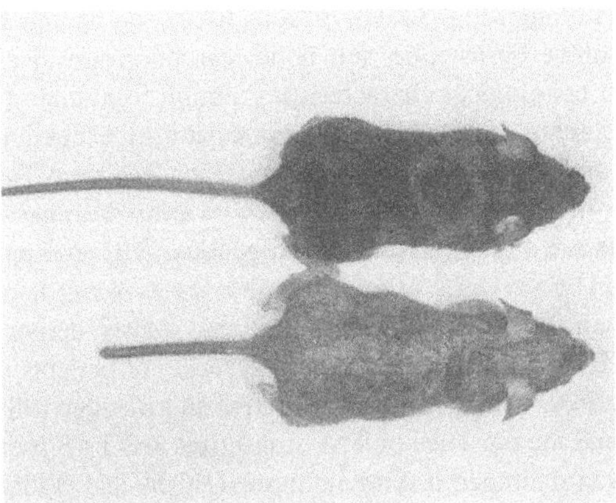

Fig. 2. Macroscopic appearance of a normal control (*top*) and a TNF-gl transgenic mouse (*bottom*) showing the resulting hair growth defect. Similar hair growth deficiency is observed in several other huTNF transgenic lines, irrespective of the gene construct used for microinjection

TNF bioactivity was undetectable in the serum of these mice when measured by standard L929 cytotoxicity assays.

5.6 A Predictable Transgenic Model of huTNF Triggered Arthritis

We have recently reported (Keffer et al. 1991) that transgenic mice carrying and expressing the 3'-modified, TNF-globin hybrid transgene develop chronic inflammatory polyarthritis with 100% phenotypic penetrance. Histological examination of most other tissues did not reveal further abnormalities. Development of arthritis in these transgenic mice can be completely suppressed by treatment with antibodies against huTNF (provided by Celltech, UK), confirming that the pathology observed is effected by the in vivo deregulated production of huTNF protein. One of these transgenic lines (Tg197), which we were able to establish and reproduce, develops macroscopic signs of disease (swelling of the ankle joints) at 3–4 weeks of age. At the same time progressive hyperplasia of the synovial layer and inflammatory infiltrates of the synovial space are evident in nearly all joints, starting from 3 weeks of age (Fig. 3A,B). Fibrous tissue and pannus formation, articular cartilage destruction and bone resorption are also observed (Fig. 3C), all histological characteristics similar to human rheumatoid arthritis (Trentham 1982). Notably, expression of exogenous huTNF mRNA was undetectable in peritoneal macrophages from Tg197 mice. Furthermore, in situ hybridization analysis of arthritic joints shows that synovial cells are a major source of exogenous TNF production (to be published). In some cases articular chondrocytes were also found to express human TNF mRNA. Several recent studies demonstrate the presence of TNF in the synovial fluid and serum of patients with rheumatoid arthritis (Saxne et al. 1988; Hopkins and Meager 1988; Yocum et al. 1989) and the presence of TNF transcripts and TNF protein in the stromal cells of rheumatoid synovial tissue (Husby and Williams 1988; Buchan et al. 1988; Macnaul et al. 1990). These findings emphasize the important role of TNF in the inflammatory processes underlying rheumatoid arthritis. In light of the fact that the histological lesions and the localization of TNF mRNA in the synovial tissue of the TNF transgenic mice are identical to the analogous characteristics of human

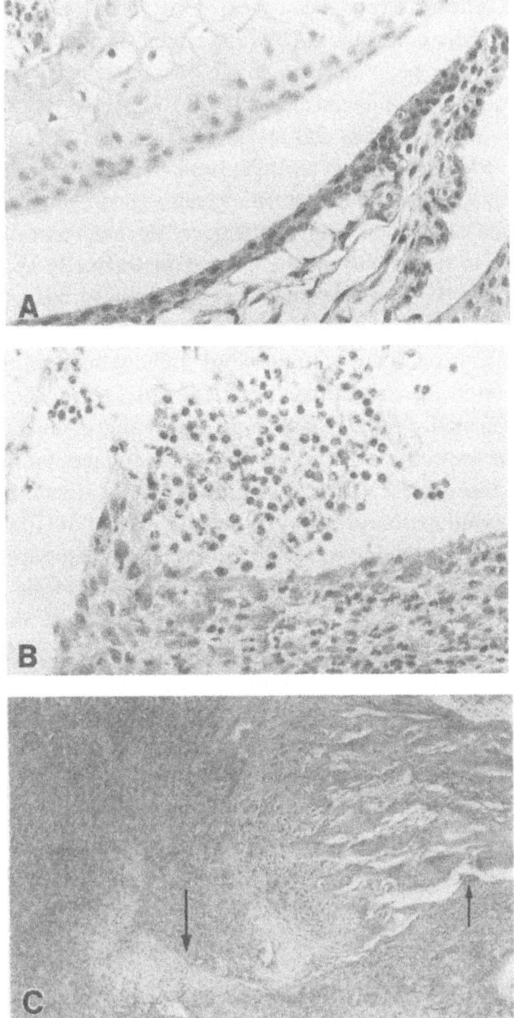

Fig. 3A–C. Progression of arthritis in the joints of a TNF-globin transgenic line. **A** Onset of synovial thickening in the knee joint of a 4-week-old transgenic mouse. **B** Accumulation of polymorphonuclear cells and lymphocytes in the knee joint synovial space of a 9-week-old mouse. **C** Fibrous tissue formation, synovial hyperplasia and pannus eroding both cartilage (*long arrow*) and bone (*short arrow*) in the ankle joint of a 4-week-old mouse

rheumatoid arthritis, it may be suggested that TNF transgenic mice developing arthritis constitute a relevant model of human arthritis. The 100% phenotypic penetrance in this model, unique amongst several other experimentally induced (Jasin 1988; Ridge et al. 1988a,b; Taurog et al. 1988; Wooley 1988) and spontaneous models of human arthritis (Hang et al. 1982; Hammer et al. 1990; Iwakura et al. 1991), should facilitate further experimentation on its pathogenesis and treatment.

The mode of deregulation that triggers development of this complex disease in transgenic mice can be experimentally approached at different levels. First, a quantitative perturbation in the expression of TNF resulting from the introduced 3'-modification, may be considered. This is consistent with previous findings supporting a role for this 3'-region in the translational efficiency of TNF mRNA (Kruys et al. 1989; Han et al. 1990). Furthermore, qualitative disturbances (i.e altered cell type specific expression) may act as triggers for the development of disease. In each case, TNF action may be direct, for example by driving proliferation of synovial cells (Butler et al. 1988; Gitter et al. 1989) and contributing to local chronic inflammatory processes, or indirect, possibly by interfering with immune homeostasis in the joint space. Backcrossing of Tg197 mice to immunodeficient mouse strains might provide insight to the latter. Finally, it may be argued that a cause in the development of arthritis in these mice is a disturbance in the ability of the membrane-bound and soluble mouse TNF receptors to modulate human TNF activities, in the light of evidence suggesting that one of the two mouse TNF receptors, the p75 TNF-R, is unable to mediate signalling through the huTNF protein. It will thus be very important to assess whether the same pathology will evolve by the use of a similar mouse TNF transgene. We are currently investigating all these possibilities.

5.7 T Cell-Targeted huTNF Expression in Transgenic Mice: Differential Localized and Systemic Activities

The biological potential of high-level, T cell-targeted expression of the human TNF gene was investigated in transgenic mice by the use of wild-type or 3'-modified huTNF gene constructs placed under the control of the T cell-specific locus control region of the human CD2 gene

(Greaves et al. 1989). HuTNF mRNA was found to be expressed exclusively in the thymus, lymph nodes and spleen of transgenic mice. Immunochemical analysis of transgenic thymocytes revealed that bioactive exogenous huTNF was produced in both the membrane-associated (26-kDa) and the secreted (17-kDa) molecular forms.

Mice expressing constitutively high levels of exogenous TNF mRNA in the T cell compartment developed within the first week after birth marked localized changes in their lymphoid organs. Thymi were obviously hypoplastic (cellularity was found to be 50-fold lower than in normal age-matched controls), depleted of lymphocytes and with a much reduced or nonexistent cortex (Fig. 4). Histology of spleen and mesenteric lymph nodes showed a perturbed structure characterized by an overall depletion of lymphocytes and an absence of germinal centers and distinct B and T cell regions. At later stages (4–5 weeks of age), these transgenic mice developed a lethal wasting syndrome associated with widespread vascular thrombosis and extensive necrosis in organs such as liver (Fig. 5), pancreas and lymph nodes. Serum TNF levels were measured to be at the level of 100–1300 pg/ml and 0.01–7 U/ml as determined by ELISA and L929 cytotoxicity assay, respectively. Administration of neutralizing anti-TNF antibodies (provided by Celltech, UK) prevented development of disease if given from birth or reversed it if given early after the onset of illness. Localized, lymphoid organ abnormalities were not always paralleled by systemic pathology. For example, in one line of mice expressing the CD2-TNF gene construct, despite pronounced lymphoid organ defects, systemic pathology never developed.

It has been previously suggested (Perez et al. 1990; Liu et al. 1989; Peck et al. 1989) that part of the complex physiology of TNF can be attributed to its differential presentation as a membrane-associated or as a secreted molecule. For example, it has been proposed that the membrane-associated 26-kDa form of TNF mediates contact-dependent or paracrine responses, in contrast to the systemic bioactivity of the secretory 17-kDa form. Transgenic mice constitutively expressing TNF in the T cell compartment offer a unique in vivo system by which to analyse the contribution of the different molecular forms of TNF in the development of localized and systemic TNF-mediated pathology. For example, this transgenic system will be useful in the evaluation of the in vivo bioactivity of nonsecretable mutant forms of TNF such as

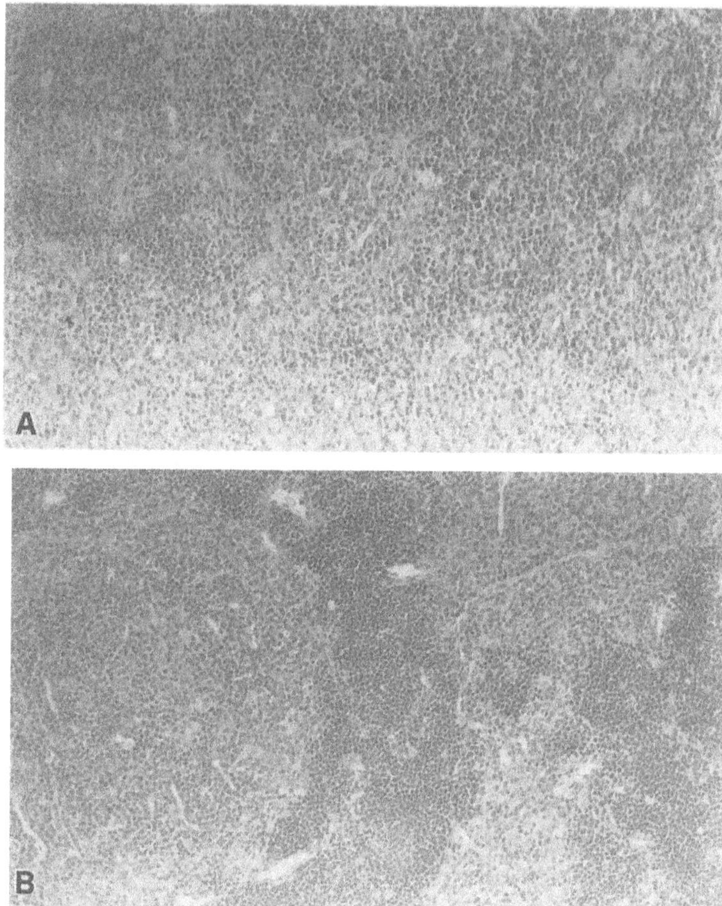

Fig. 4. A Thymus from a Tg7 CD2-TNF transgenic mouse at 3.5 weeks of age, showing the depletion of lymphocytes and the absence of a densely packed, definable cortex area. **B** Normal thymus histology in the nonaffected Tg90 CD2-TNF transgenic mouse line. Tg90 mice were found to express very low levels of exogenous human TNF mRNA and did not develop abnormalities in their lymphoid organs

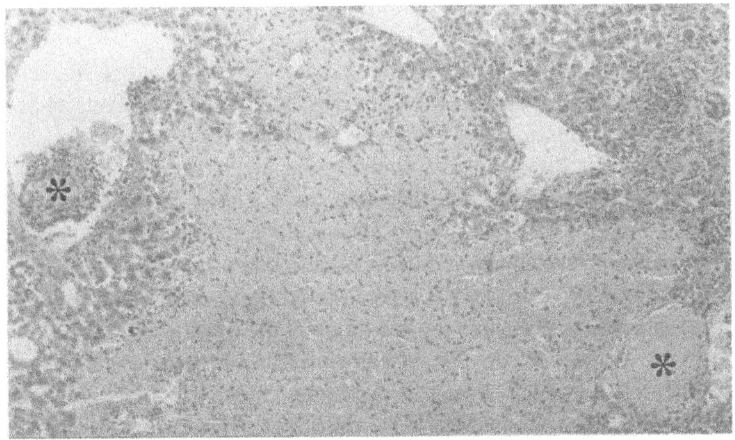

Fig. 5. Ischaemic necrosis of liver tissue in a Tg211 CD2-TNF-globin transgenic mouse containing two vessels which are occluded by large thrombi (*asterisks*)

those described by Perez et al. (1990). Finally, given the species specific nature of the mouse p75 TNF receptor it may be assumed that the pathology induced in these transgenic mice is associated exclusively with p55 TNF receptor signalling. Conceivably, the differential contribution of each of the two TNF receptors in TNF mediated disease can be assessed by comparison of the biological potential of human versus mouse TNF in the transgenic systems developed.

5.8 Concluding Remarks

We have established several transgenic mouse lines carrying and expressing wild-type and modified human TNF transgenes and have been able to demonstrate the following:

1. We have shown that endotoxin-responsive expression of human TNF transgenes can be established in transgenic mice and that the

necessary *cis*-acting DNA information for this is contained within a 3.6-kb DNA fragment.
2. Using 3'-modified transgenes we obtained evidence suggesting that the 3'-region of the human TNF gene is necessary for macrophage specific expression.
3. We provide direct in vivo evidence for a role for TNF in the pathogenesis of arthritis. Furthermore, we can show that development of arthritis in the TNF transgenic mice can be prevented by the in vivo administration of monoclonal antibodies to human TNF. This or other inhibitors of TNF action should prove useful in the design of therapeutic protocols for this group of diseases.
4. T cell-targeted production of human TNF in transgenic mice leads to local (lymphoid organ) and systemic (wasting, ischaemia) toxic effects. The transgenic system which was developed demonstrates the important role of T cell-specific TNF production in the development of specific pathology and is expected to facilitate further molecular characterization of TNF action.

TNF occupies a dominant role in the pathophysiology of a seemingly diverse range of diseases. The understanding of its pleiotropic actions necessitates the analysis of the mechanisms regulating TNF and TNF receptor production and functional potency. The use of transgenic mice to pursue this aim will provide useful information about how this complex processes are regulated and will also provide excellent models of human diseases and clinical disorders for testing new therapies and pharmacological approaches to their treatment.

Acknowledgements. I thank my colleagues, past and present, for practical work, discussions and ideas.

References

Beutler B, Cerami A (1989) The biology of cachectin/TNF- a primary mediator of the host response. Ann Rev Immunol 7:625–655
Beutler B, Krochin N, Milsark IW, Luedke C, Cerami A (1986) Control of cachectin (tumor necrosis factor) synthesis: mechanisms of endotoxin resistance. Science 232:977–980

Brockhaus M, Schoenfeld HJ, Schlaeger EJ, Hunziker W, Lesslauer W, Loetcher H (1990) Identification of two types of tumor necrosis factor receptors on human cell lines by monoclonal antibodies. Proc Natl Acad Sci USA 87:3127–3131

Buchan G, Barrett K, Turner M, Chantry D, Maini RN, Feldmann M (1988) Interleukin-1 and tumour necrosis factor mRNA expression in rheumatoid arthritis: prolonged production of IL-1α. Clin Exp Immunol 73:449–455

Butler DM, Piccoli DS, Hart PH, Hamilton JA (1988) Stimulation of human synovial fibroblast DNA synthesis by recombinant human cytokines. J Rheumatology 15:1463–1470

Caput D, Beutler B, Hartog K, Thayer R, Shimer SB, Cerami A (1986) Identification of a common nucleotide sequence in the 3'-untranslated region of mRNA molecules specifying inflammatory mediators. Proc Natl Acad Sci USA 83:1670–1674

Carswell E, Old L, Cassel R, Green S, Fiore N, Williamson B (1975) An endotoxin serum factor that causes necrosis of tumours. Proc Natl Acad Sci USA 72:3666

Engelman H, Aderka D, Rubinstein M, Rotman D, Wallach D (1989) A tumor necrosis factor-binding protein purified to homogeneity from human urine protects cells from tumor necrosis factor toxicity. J Biol Chem 264:11974–11980

Esparza I, Mannel D, Ruppel A, Falk W, Krammer PH (1987) Interferon-gamma (IFN-γ) and lymphotoxin (LT) or tumor necrosis factor (TNF) synergize to activate macrophages for tumoricidal and schistosomulicidal functions. Lymphokine Res 6:1715.

Gamble JR, Harlan JM, Klebanoff SJ, Lopez AF, Vadas MA (1985) Stimulation of the adherence of neutrophils to umbilical vein endothelium by human recombinant tumor necrosis factor. Proc Natl Acad Sci USA 82:8667–8671

Gitter BD, Labus JM, Lees SL, Scheetz ME (1989) Characteristics of human synovial fibroblast activation by IL-1β and TNFα. Immunology 66:196–200

Grau GE, Piguet PF, Vassali P, Lambert P-H (1989) Tumor necrosis factor and other cytokines in cerebral malaria: experimental and clinical data. Immunol 112:49–70

Greaves DR, Wilson FD, Lang G, Kioussis D (1989) Human CD2 3'-flanking sequences confer high-level, T cell specific, position independent gene expression in transgenic mice. Cell 56:979–986

Hammer RE, Malka SD, Richardson JA, Tang JP, Taurog JD (1990) Spontaneous inflammatory disease in transgenic rats expressing HLA-B27 and human β_2m: an animal model of HLA-B27-associated human disorders. Cell 63:1099–1112

Han J, Brown T, Beutler B (1990) Endotoxin-responsive sequences control cachectin/tumor necrosis factor at the translational level. J Exp Med 171:465–475

Hang LM, Theofilopoulos AN, Dixon FJ (1982) A spontaneous rheumatoid arthritis-like disease in MRL/l mice. J Exp Med 155:1690–1701

Held W, MacDonald HR, Weissman IL, Hess MW, Mueller C (1990) Genes encoding tumor necrosis factor α and granzyme A are expressed during development of autoimmune diabetes. Proc Natl Acad Sci USA 7:2239–2243

Husby G, Williams RC Jr (1988) Synovial localization of tumor necrosis factor in patients with rheumatoid arthritis. J Autoimmun 1:363–371

Iwakura Y, Tosu M, Yoshida E, Takiguchi M, Sato K, Kitajima I, Nishioka K, Yamamoto K, Takeda T, Hatanaka M, Yamamoto H, Sekiguchi T (1991) Induction of inflammatory arthropathy resembling rheumatoid arthritis in mice transgenic for HTLV-I. Science 253:1026–1028

Jasin HE (1988) Chronic arthritis in rabbits. Meth Enzymol 162:379–385

Jue DM, Sherry B, Luedke C, Manogue KR, Cerami A (1990) Processing of newly synthesized cachectin/tumor necrosis factor in endotoxin stimulated macrophages. Biochemistry 29:8371–8377

Keffer, Probert L, Cazlaris H, Georgopoulos S, Kaslaris E, Kioussis D, Kollias G (1991) Transgenic mice expressing human tumor necrosis factor: a predictive genetic model of arthritis. EMBO J 13:4025–4031

Kinkhabwala M, Sehajpal P, Skolnik E, Smith D, Sharma VK, Vlassara H, Cerami A, Suthanthiran M (1990) A novel addition to the T cell repertory; cell surface expression of tumor necrosis factor/cachectin by activated normal human T cells. J Exp Med 171:941–946

Kohno T, Brewer MT, Baker SL, Schwartz PE, King MW, Hale KK, Squires CH, Thompson RC, Vannice JL (1990) A second tumor necrosis factor receptor gene product can shed a naturally occuring tumor necrosis factor inhibitor. Proc Natl Acad Sci USA 87:8331–8335

Kriegler M, Perez C, DeFay K, Albert I, Lu SD (1988) A novel form of TNF/cachectin is a cell surface cytotoxic transmembrane protein: Ramifications for the complex physiology of TNF. Cell 53:45–53

Kruys V, Matinx O, Shaw G, Deschamps J, Huez G (1989) Translational blockade imposed by cytokine-derived UA-rich sequences. Science 245:852–855

Lewis M, Tartaglia TA, Lee A, Bennett GL, Rice GC, Wong GHW, Chen EY, Goeddel DV (1991) Cloning and expression of cDNAs for two distinct murine tumor necrosis factor receptors demonstrate one receptor is species specific. Proc Natl Acad Sci USA 88:2830–2834

Liu CC, Detmers PA, Jiang S, Young JD-E (1989) Identification and characterization of a membrane-bound cytotoxin of murine cytolytic lymphocytes that is related to tumor necrosis factor/cachectin. Proc Natl Acad Sci USA 86:3286–3290

Luettig B, Decker T, Lohmann-Matthes ML (1989) Evidence for the existence of two forms of membrane tumor necrosis factor: an integral protein and a molecule attached to its receptor. J Immunol 143:4034–4038

Macnaul KL, Hutchinson NI, Parsons JN, Bayne EK, Tocci MJ (1990) Analysis of IL-1 and TNF-α gene expression in human rheumatoid synoviocytes and normal monocytes by in situ hybridization. J Immunol 145:4154–4166

Nawroth PP, Stern DM (1986) Modulation of endothelial cell hemostatic properties by tumor necrosis factor. J Exp Med 163:740–745

Old LJ (1990) Tumor necrosis factor. In: Bonavida B, Granger G (eds) Tumor Necrosis Factor: Structure, Mechanism of Action, Role in Disease and Therapy. Basel, Karger, pp 1–30

Oliff A, Defeo-Jones D, Boyer M, Martinez D, Kiefer D, Vuocolo G, Wolfe A, Socher SH (1987) Tumors secreting human TNF/cachectin induce cachexia in mice. Cell 50:555–563

Osborn L, Kunkel S, Nabel GJ (1989) Tumor necrosis factor α and interleukin 1 stimulate the human immunodeficiency virus enhancer by activation of the nuclear factor κB. Proc Natl Acad Sci USA 86:2336–2340

Peck R, Brockhaus M, Frey JR (1989) Cell surface tumor necrosis factor (TNF) acounts for monocyte- and lymphocyte- mediated killing of TNF-resistant target cells. Cell Immunol 122:1–10

Perez C, Albert I, DeFay K, Zachariades N, Gooding L, Kriegler M (1990) A non-secretable cell surface mutant of tumour necrosis factor (TNF) kills by cell to cell contact. Cell 63:251–258

Piguet PF, Grau GE, Allet B, Vassalli P (1987) Tumor necrosis factor/cachectin is an effector of skin and gut lesions of the acute phase of graft-vs.-host disease. J Exp Med 166:1280–1289

Porteu F, Nathan C (1990) Shedding of tumor necrosis factor receptors by activated human neutrophils. J Exp Med 172:599–607

Ranges GE, Zlotnik A, Espevik T, Dinarello CA, Cerami A, Palladino MAJr (1988) Tumor necrosis factor α/cachectin is a growth factor for thymocytes. J Exp Med 167:1472–1478

Ridge SC, Oronsky AL, Kerwar SS (1988a) Type II collagen-induced arthritis in rats. Meth Enzymol 162:355–360

Ridge SC, Zabriskie JB, Oronsky AL, Kerwar SS (1988b) Streptococcal cell wall-induced arthritis in rats. Meth Enzymol 162:373–379

Saxne T, Palladino MA Jr, Heinegard D, Talal N, Wollheim FA (1988) Detection of tumor necrosis factor α but not tumor necrosis factor β in rheumatoid arthritis synovial fluid and serum. Arthritis and Rheumatism 31:1041–1045

Seckinger P, Isaaz S, Dayer JM (1989) Purification and biologic characterization of a specific tumor necrosis factor-α inhibitor. J Biol Chem 264:11966–11973

Semb H, Peterson J, Tavernier J, Olivecrona T (1987)Multiple effects of tumor necrosis factor on lipoprotein lipase in vivo. J Biol Chem 262:8390–8394

Shalaby MR, Espevic T, Rice GC, Ammann AJ, Figari IS, Ranges GE, Palladino MAJr (1988) The involvement of human tumor necrosis factors-α and -β in the mixed lymphocyte reaction. J Immunol 141:499–503

Shaw G, Kamen R (1986) A conserved AU sequence from the 3'-untranslated region of GM-CSF mRNA mediates selective mRNA degradation. Cell 46:659–667

Smith R, Baglioni C (1989) Multimeric structure of the tumor necrosis factor receptor of HeLa cells. J Biol Chem 264:14646–14652

Tartaglia LA, Weber RF, Figari IS, Reynolds C, Palladino MA, Goeddel DV (1991) The two different receptors for tumor necrosis factor mediate distinct cellular responses. Proc Natl Acad Sci USA 88:9292–9296

Taurog JD, Argentiery DC, McReynolds RA (1988) Adjuvant arthritis. Meth Enzymol 162:339–355

Tracey KJ, Beutler B, Lowry SF, Merryweather J, Wolpe S, Milsark IW, Hariri RJ, Fahey III TJ, Zentella A, Albert JD, Shires GT, Cerami A (1986) Shock and tissue injury induced by recombinant human cachectin. Science 234:470–474

Trentham DE (1982) Collagen arthritis as a relevant model for rheumatoid arthritis. Arthr. Rheumatism 25:911–915

Vilcek J, Palombella VJ, Henriksen-DeStefano D, Swenson C, Feinman R, Hirai M, Tsujimoto M (1986) Fibroblast growth enhancing activity of tumor necrosis factor and its relationship to other polypeptide growth factors. J Exp Med 163:632–643

Wooley PH (1988) Collagen-induced arthritis in the mouse. Meth Enzymol 162:361–373

Yocum DE, Esparza L, Dubry S, Benjamin JB, Volz R, Scuderi P (1989) Characteristics of tumor necrosis factor production in rheumatoid arthritis. Cellular Immunol 122:131–145

6 Mammary Neoplasia in Mouse Mammary Tumor Virus-Transforming Growth Factor α Transgenic Mice

Robert J. Coffey and Peter J. Dempsey

6.1 Introduction

In this chapter we discuss our experience with mammary neoplasia in mouse mammary tumor virus-transforming growth factor α (MMTV-TGFα) transgenic mice. Before doing this, recent advances in the study of TGFα will be reviewed and placed into the context of epidermal growth factor (EGF) and other EGF-like molecules with special emphasis on the mammary gland. This review is not intended to be comprehensive, and, in part, will be highly speculative.

6.2 Background

6.2.1 Discovery of Transforming Growth Factors

TGFα originally was isolated from conditioned medium of virally transformed 3T3 cells [21] and later from conditioned medium of human carcinoma cells [66]. Addition of this partially purified material to normal fibroblasts caused the reversible appearance of a malignant (transformed) phenotype. Consequently, the protein was named transforming growth factor. Later it was shown that this transforming activity was comprised of two distinct proteins, now designated TGFα and TGFβ [54]. It was initially postulated that TGFα acted in an autocrine manner to induce a malignant phenotype. According to this hypothesis, TGFα secreted by the malignant cell binds to specific EGF receptors on the cell surface and promotes proliferation, thus conferring a growth advantage to this cell over its nontransformed neighbors [64]. Since TGFα was also observed in embryonic cells and tissues [68, 75], it was suggested that TGFα was an embryonic growth factor inappropriately expressed in neoplasia.

6.2.2 Structure of the TGFα Gene and Protein

The human TGFα gene spans 70-100 kb on chromosome 2 and contains six exons [22, 24]. The 4.5–4.8 kb TGFα mRNA transcript encodes a 160-amino acid peptide which is schematically depicted in Fig. 1. A signal peptide in the amino terminus is presumably cleaved prior to exit from the cell. N- and 0-linked glycosylation sites are indicated by the asterisks. The 50-amino acid polypeptide is produced by proteolytic cleavage of the ALA VAL VAL residues that flank either end of the mature molecule. Six cysteine residues in the mature peptide form three disulfide bridges. There is a hydrophobic transmembrane region followed by an intracellular cystoplasmic tail with seven cysteine residues, some of which are covalently linked to palmitate [10].

The reported sizes of the TGFα protein range from 5 to 26 kDa. This variation may reflect differential glycosylation and proteolytic cleavage, as well as dimerization and the presence of binding proteins. Possible distinct biological roles of higher molecular weight forms of

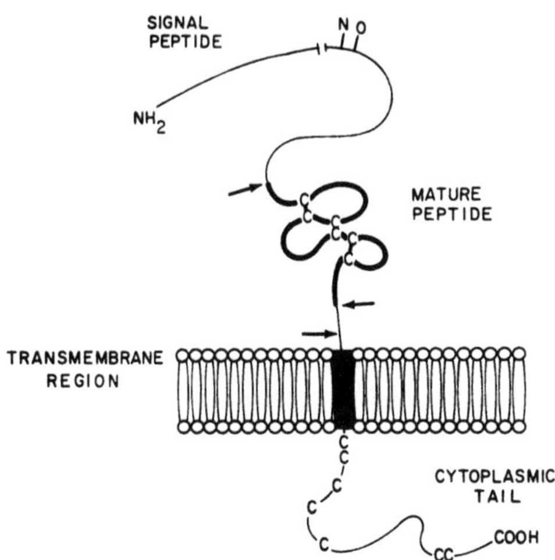

Fig. 1. Scheme of TGFα peptide. *Arrows* indicate sites of proteolytic cleavage

TGFα have not been explored. In a number of TGFα-expressing cell lines, the protein is detected in cell extracts, but not in the conditioned medium [23]. The biological significance of this observation has been explored in parallel by two independent groups [9, 76]. The arrows in Fig. 1 indicate sites of mutation engineered by these investigators that result in membrane fixation of TGFα. These mutated forms of TGFα are able to activate EGF receptors on neighboring cells. This observation has important implications for the actions of TGFα, e.g., this cell–cell stimulation ("juxtacrine" stimulation) might play a role in developmental processes that depend on discrete cell–cell interactions, or it might target pro-TGFα expressing cells to tissue sites rich in EGFR [44, 50]. There is increasing evidence that local production/processing of TGFα may confer biological consequences distinct from systemic delivery/exogenous administration of the growth factor [37].

6.2.3 The EGF/TGFα Receptor

There is 35 % structural identity between TGFα and EGF; however, all six cysteine residues are conserved and formation of three disulfide bridges imparts sufficient structural identity for both peptides to bind to the EGFR. The EGFR is a 170 kDa protein that consists of a cell surface ligand receptor domain, a single hydrophobic transmembrane segment and a highly conserved cytoplasmic tyrosine kinase domain [12]. Binding of EGF or TGFα to the receptor initiates a complex program of activation of intrinsic kinase activity, increases in cytosolic calcium, and ultimately DNA synthesis and cellular growth. In addition, clustering and dimerization of receptors occurs with binding of ligand to cell surface receptor followed by internalization and degradation of the ligand/receptor complexes within lysosomes. A 65-amino acid cytoplasmic stretch of the EGFR has been identified that mediates the increase in cytoplasmic calcium and ligand/receptor internalization (the CAIN domain) [14]. Activation of the EGFR tyrosine kinase appears to be necessary for subsequent biological activity. An active area of research is identification of substrates for this tyrosine kinase; activation of phospholipase C-γ 1 appears to be a promising candidate [71, 72].

6.2.4 Cellular Distribution of TGFα

TGFα expression is clearly not restricted to the embryonic and neoplastic state. We were the first to demonstrate that TGFα is produced in vitro and in vivo by a nontransformed epithelial cell, human keratinocytes [16]. Subsequently, production of TGFα has been detected in a wide range of normal cells and tissues, including mammary epithelium [40, 62], activated macrophages [41] and gastrointestinal tissues [13, 42, 43, 5, 3, 65].

It should be noted that the examples cited above represent cells and tissues in which TGFα mRNA, as well as protein, have been detected, thus reflecting true local synthesis rather than delivery from a remote site. Since EGF is expressed by a selective population of normal cells and tissues (eg, salivary gland, Brunner's gland, kidney), the widespread production of TGFα has led us to suggest that in vivo TGFα, and not EGF, is the major ligand for the EGFR. This statement must be qualified by certain caveats. First, Wright's group has demonstrated that a novel cell lineage produces EGF in the chronically injured gastrointestinal tract [77]. Second, additional members of the EGF/TGFα family have been identified (see below), and certain of these ligands may be as widely expressed as TGFα.

6.2.5 Family of TGFα/EGF Ligands and Receptors

Fig. 2 lists the family of TGFα ligands and receptors. EGF and EGFR were the first to be characterized (see [12] for review). Two additional receptors with homology to EGFR have been identified, erbB-2 and erbB-3 [57, 38]. Overexpression of c-erbB-2 directly correlates with prognosis in patients with breast cancer [7, 61]. Of interest, a 44-kDa glycoprotein designated neu differentiation factor (NDF) has been purified to homogeneity from ras-transformed rat cells and appears to be a ligand for erbB-2 [51, 74]; this may be the rat homologue of a 45-kDa protein heregulin-α that has been purified from the conditioned medium of a human breast cancer cell line (MDA-MB-231), cloned and sequenced [34]. Addition of NDF to mammary epithelial cells results in a differentiated phenotype [51]. No ligand for erbB-3 has been identified thus far.

There is an expanding number of members of the TGFα family of ligands. These share structural similarities, including the conservation of 6 cysteines of the EGF motif which, in EGF, are involved in the three disulfide bonds defining the tertiary structure and conferring the ability to bind the EGFR. With the exception of cripto (for which recombinant peptide is not yet available), these family members have been shown to bind the EGFR. The best characterized of these ligands are EGF, TGFα and amphiregulin (AR), whose protein structures are shown in Fig. 3 . The disulfide bonds formed between cysteines 1 and 3, 2 and 4, and 5 and 6 result in formation of three loops that provide the backbone structure to these molecules. AR was initially cloned from 12-0-tetradecanoylphorbol-13-acetate (TPA)-induced MCF-7 cells [60, 53]; more recently it has been isolated from conditioned medium of human keratinocytes [19] in which, like TGFα, it appears to act as an autocrine growth factor. Newer members of the EGF/TGFα

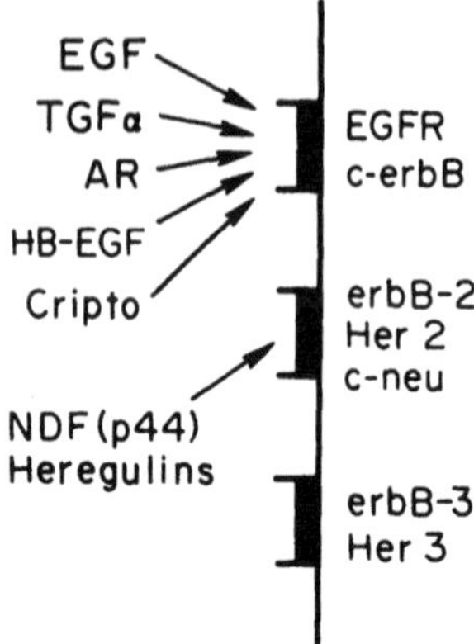

Fig. 2. Family of TGFα ligands and receptors

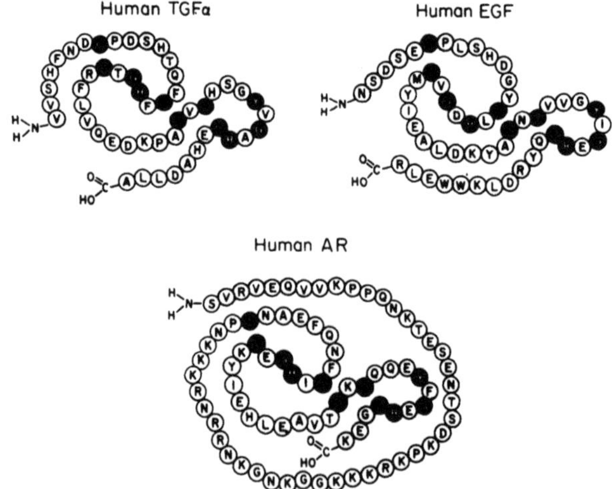

Fig. 3. Amino acid stucture of human TGFα, EGF and amphiregulin

family which have not been as well characterized include heparin bind-ing (HB)-EGF and cripto. HB-EGF was cloned from human macro-phages [33], and cripto was identified initially in a human teratocarci-noma cell line [15]. A comprehensive analysis of the pattern of expression of this family of ligands and receptors in breast cancer has not been performed.

6.2.6 Biological Actions of TGFα

The biological actions of TGFα and EGF have been reviewed recently in detail [12]. These peptides share a similar spectrum of activity since both peptides bind the same receptor. Shared properties that are of potential importance to the mammary gland include stimulation of cel-lular proliferation [12], cell migration [2, 4], angiogenesis [58], arterial blood flow [30] and fluid and electrolyte exchange [49].

6.3 TGFα in Mammary Neoplasia

6.3.1 TGFα in Mammary Gland Development

Several different experimental approaches have suggested a role for growth factors of the TGFα/EGF family in the growth and develop-ment of the mouse mammary gland. Pregnancy-like lobuloalveolar de-velopment of gland from estrogen/progesterone (E/P)-primed subadult female mice can be achieved in whole organ culture. However, the maximal morphogenetic response requires the presence of EGF in the culture medium [67, 69]. Crude extracts of mammary-derived growth factor (MDGF), which binds to EGF receptors but is immunologically distinct from EGF, can substitute for EGF in this culture system [69].

In vivo experiments using slow-release pellets inserted directly into the mammary gland provide direct evidence that EGF and TGFα can stimulate local lobuloalveolar development, although systemic delivery of estrogen and progesterone was required in the case of EGF [70]. In these experiments, TGFα was effective at one-fifth the level required for EGF [70]. In ovariectomized mice, EGF alone induced local ductal morphogenesis, although not lobuloalveolar development [17]. Similarly, Snedeker et al. [63] have shown implanation of pellets containing either EGF or TGFα into the regressed mammary gland of ovariectomized mice can stimulate the reappearance of end buds. In contrast, administration of relatively high doses of EGF caused inhibition of mouse mammary ductal morphogenesis [18].

Snedeker et al. [63] have demonstrated the expression of EGF and TGFα mRNA transcripts in the normal mouse mammary gland. More importantly, differences between the mRNA levels of EGF and TGFα were observed during the development and differentiation of the mammary gland (e.g., lactation). Immunolocalization of EGF and TGFα in the mammary gland has also shown different cellular localization of each polypeptide within the mammary epithelium [63]. TGFα colocalizes with EGFR to the proliferative terminal end bud compartment, whereas EGF resides at the luminal surface where it might play a role in fluid transport and/or milk secretion. Together, these data suggest that EGF and TGFα may play different roles in normal mammary gland morphogenesis.

Further insight into the effect of TGFα on the mammary gland development has been achieved by overexpression of TGFα in transgenic mice under the control of either MMTV [45] and mouse metallothionein [36, 56] promoters. Preliminary data from Jhappan et al. [36] has revealed that penetration of the ductal epithelium into the mesenchymal fat pad was impeded in adolescent mice at 6 weeks. By 12 weeks of age, both the transgenic and nontransgenic fat pads were completely filled. At 7 weeks of age the transgenic mammary gland had a denser network of branching ducts and ductules and significant increase in DNA synthesis was observed in the mammary epithelium which was not restricted to the end bud region but also included large number of cells in subtending ducts. Sandgren et al. [56] have observed increased ductal and alveolar secretions in the transgenic mammary glands.

6.3.2 Features of Mammary Neoplasia in MMTV-TGFα Transgenic Mice

There has been contradictory in vitro data as to the role of TGFα in malignant transformation. Transfection of TGFα cDNA constructs into nontransformed Rat-1 fibroblasts resulted in a transformed phenotype that was reversed by the addition of antibodies to TGFα [55]. However, NIH 3T3 cells transfected with similar TGFα constructs did not exhibit features of transformation [29]. Additional uncertainty as to the role of TGFα in neoplasia arose from the observation that TGFα is produced in a wide range of normal cells and tissues, including mammary epithelium [40, 62].

To better understand the role of TGFα in the development of neoplasia, three groups have examined the consequences of overproduction of TGFα in mice bearing a TGFα cDNA transgene under control of MMTV, metallothionein 1 (MT) and elastase promoters [45, 36, 56]. Mammary adenocarcinoma was observed in postlactational female mice under control of the MMTV and MT promoter. In the report of Jhappan et al. [36], hepatic neoplasia also occurred and was more frequent than mammary carcinoma. In the MT-TGFα transgenic mice [36, 56], breast cancer developed despite low expression of the transgene in the mammary gland relative to other tissues (liver, kidney, gut). These findings suggest that mammary epithelium is particularly susceptible to development of neoplasia in the setting of enhanced TGFα production and that in this in vivo model TGFα acts as an oncogene.

Eight independent lines have been established from injection of the MMTV-TGFα construct into fertilized mouse eggs [45, 31]. The transgene is expressed in the mammary gland, salivary gland and male reproductive tissues. One line (254) exhibits overexpression of the transgene in the skin and has developed generalized sebaceous gland hyperplasia. Expression of the transgene begins as early as 3 weeks of age and precedes any histological changes. The major histological abnormalities have been confined to the mammary gland; no phenotypic abnormalities have been identified in the male seminal vesicles and testes despite high levels of transgene expression in these tissues. Within the mammary gland, overexpression of TGFα is restricted to the mammary epithelium, as confirmed by in situ hybridization and immunohistochemistry. A range of histological abnormalities is seen in the mammary gland: cystic and solid hyperplasia, dysplasia, adenoma and adenocarcinoma. Four of the 8 lines have developed mammary adenocarcinoma. In the best studied line (line 29), 65 % of multiparous mice and 45% of virgin mice develop hyperplasia by 12 months of age; by 16 months of age, 40 % of multiparous mice and 30% of virgin mice develop adenocarcinoma.

How does enhanced production of TGFα lead to mammary neoplasia? Clearly, TGFα is a mitogen for mammary epithelium. Proliferation of normal mammary epithelial cell lines is stimulated by TGFα in vitro [62] and local application of TGFα in slow-release form to mammary glands of 5-week-old mice is associated with local alveolar and ductal growth [70]. In vivo, DNA synthesis is enhanced in the mammary glands of MT-TGFα transgenic mice [36]. However, overproduction of TGFα by itself appears insufficient to cause mammary neoplasia and additional events are necessary [45]. One such event may be upregulation of EGF receptor. Recent in vitro transfection studies indicate that marked up regulation of TGFα production may contribute to neoplasia if sufficient numbers of EGFR are present [25, 26, 59, 46], and it has been suggested that an abundance of both ligand and its cognate receptor is required to achieve a critical threshold in terms of the mitogenic signal cascade to induce a malignant phenotype [25]. In human tumors, overexpression of the EGF receptor has been reported in mammary carcinoma and squamous cell carcinoma of the head and neck [32, 78]. In this context, we have shown that mammary tissues harboring histologic abnormalities express high levels of the TGFα transgene and display increased expression of the endogenous EGFR mRNA [45].

Nonetheless this does not provide a mechanism by which overproduction of TGFα leads to neoplasia. Based on a review of the literature and preliminary data that we have generated, we propose that TGFα, when sufficiently overproduced, may act as a tumor promoter.

6.3.3 TGFα/EGF as Tumor Promoters
in Mammary Carcinogenesis

Carcinogenesis is a complex, multistep process that has been divided into multiple discernible stages, including initiation, promotion and progression; in these likely overlapping stages, environmental and endogenous factors act through a variety of different biochemical and genetic mechanisms [8, 73, 79]. In vivo studies in mice have provided circumstantial evidence that EGF contributes to mammary neoplasia.

In a strain of mice with a high incidence of spontaneous mammary carcinoma (C3H), sialoadenectomized virgin females had a nearly fivefold decrease in the incidence of mammary tumors at 52 weeks, compared to sham-operated controls (12.8 % vs 62.5 %) [39]. Sialoadenectomy is thought to mediate its effects by depleting the mouse of a major source of EGF. Administration of EGF at the time of sialoadenectomy increased the tumor incidence to 33 %. In a subsequent report, sialoadenectomized virgin females of strains also predisposed to mammary cancer had a reduced incidence of premalignant histological changes [35]. These observations, coupled with additional in vitro data, support a role for EGF as a tumor promoter.

Tumor promoters can be defined as compounds which have very weak or no carcinogenic activity when tested alone but enhance tumor formation when applied repeatedly following a low or suboptimal dose of a carcinogen (initiator) [8]. Most promoters induce proliferation in target cells, yet a number of agents which induce proliferation in specific target tissues are not active as promoters. While the precise mechanisms of action for all promoters are not understood, the likeliest common action of these agents is to cause a selective clonal expansion of the initiated cell population resulting in a clinically evident premalignant lesion and increasing the number of cells at risk for further changes in neoplastic progression [73, 11, 27, 28, 47]. A classic tumor promoter is TPA. The discovery that TPA binds and activates the enzyme protein kinase C (PKC) has revealed common molecular mechanisms for growth factor activity, signal transduction and activation of specific cancer genes (oncogenes).

In this context, TPA and EGF mediate similar effects. Both agents activate PKC and downregulate the EGF receptor (although reportedly through different mechanisms; [6, 20, 48, 52]. Administration of both agents in vivo results in epidermal hyperplasia ([1]; M. Stahlman, personal communication). Based on the biochemical and functional homology between EGF and TGFα, we have demonstrated that selected effects of TPA may be mediated through enhanced production of TGFα. Administration of TPA to cultured keratinocytes results in a 20-fold induction of TGFα mRNA and protein [52]. This observation lends further support for the hypothesis that TGFα, when sufficiently overproduced, may act as a tumor promoter.

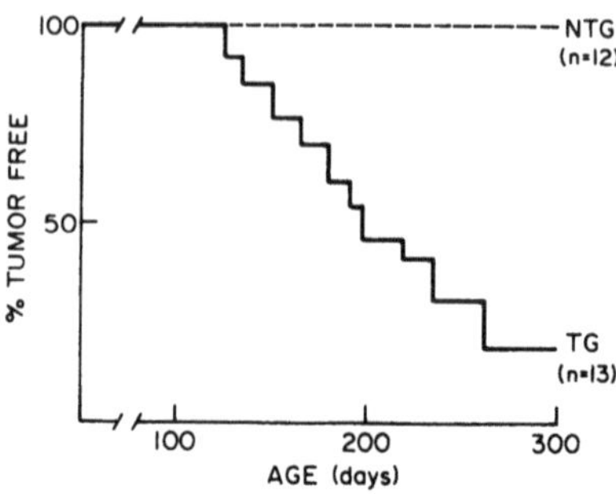

Fig. 4. Time to development of palpable mammary tumors in virgin MMTV-TGFα transgenic females treated with a single 0.5 mg orogastric dose of DMBA at 8 weeks of age

Current evidence supports the concept that TGFα may act as a tumor promoter; however, other explanations are possible. One could argue that the high levels of TGFα in the MMTV-TGFα transgenic mice have produced a population of constitutively initiated cells. Alternatively, TGFα as a mitogen may expand the population of normally proliferating cells, thus providing a larger target for subsequent initiating event(s). We cannot formally dismiss these possibilities. The latter notion and a more classical tumor-promoting action for TGFα are not mutually exclusive.

To explore the possible role of TGFα as a tumor promoter in mammary carcinogenesis, we have begun studies in which initiating doses of dimethylbenzanthracene (DMBA) have been administered to MMTV-TGFα transgenic mice and nontransgenic littermates. A single initiating dose of DMBA (0.5 mg via intragastric instillation) was administered to line 29 virgin transgenic females and their nontransgenic littermates at 8 weeks of age. It should be noted that spontaneous mammary tumors do not occur before 320 days in line 29 virgin females. To date, 10/13 transgenic mice and 0/12 nontransgenic mice have developed mammary carcinoma by 220 days of age; median age at time of tumor formation in transgenic mice was 120 days (Fig. 4). These promising results provide circumstantial evidence that overproduction of TGFα in the mammary gland may act to promote mammary tumor formation.

References

1. Argyris TS (1981) The regulation of epidermal hyperplastic growth. CRC Crit Rev Toxicol 9:151–200
2. Bade EG, Feindler S (1988) Liver epithelial cell migration induced by epidermal growth factor or transforming growth factor alpha is associated with changes in the gene expression of secreted proteins. In Vitro Cell Devel Biol 24:149–154
3. Barnard JA, Polk WH, Moses HL, Coffey RJ (1991) Production of tranforming growth factor alpha by normal rat small intestine. Am J Physiol 261:C994–C1000
4. Barrandon Y, Green H (1987) Cell migration is essential for sustained growth of keratinocyte colonies: the roles of transforming growth factor-α and epidermal growth factor. Cell 50:1131–1137
5. Beauchamp RD, Barnard JA, McCutchen CM, Cherner JA, Coffey RJ (1989) Localization of transforming growth factor-α and its receptor in gastric mucosal cells: implications for a regulatory role in acid secretion and mucosal renewal. J Clin Invest 84: 1017–1023
6. Beguinot L, Hanover JA, Ito S, Richert ND, Willingham MC, Pastan I (1985) Phorbol esters induce transient internalization without degradation of unoccupied epidermal growth factor receptors. Proc Natl Acad Sci USA 82:2774–2778
7. Berger MS, Locher GW, Sauer S, Gullick WJ, Waterfield MD, Groner B, Hynes R (1988) Correlation of c-erbB-2 gene amplification and protein expression in human breast carcinoma with nodal status and nuclear grading. Cancer Res 48:1238–1243
8. Boutwell RK (1989) Model systems for defining initiation, promotion, and progression of skin neoplasms. In: Slaga TJ et al (eds) Skin carcinogenesis: mechanisms and human relevance. Liss, New York, pp 3–15
9. Brachmann R, Lindquist PB, Nagashima M, Kohr W, Lipari T, Napier M, Derynck R (1989) Transmembrane TGF-α precursors activate EGF/TGF-α receptors. Cell 56:691–700
10. Bringman TS, Lindquist PB, Derynck R (1987) Different transforming growth factor-α species are derived from a glycosylated and palmitoylated transmembrane precursor. Cell 48:429–440
11. Burns F, Albert R, Altshuler B, Morris E (1983) Approach to risk assessment for genotoxic carcinogens based on data from the mouse skin initiation-promotion model. Environ Health Perspect 50:309–320
12. Carpenter G, Wahl MI (1990) The epidermal growth factor family. In: Sporn MB, Roberts AB (eds) Peptide growth factors and their receptors I. Springer, Berlin Heidelberg New York, pp 69–171 (Handbook of Experimental Pharmacology, vol 95)
13. Cartlidge SA, Elder JB (1989) Transforming growth factor-α and epidermal growth levels in normal human gastrointestinal mucosa. Int J Cancer 60:657–660

14. Chen WS, Lazar CS, Lund KA, Welsh JB, Chang CP, Walton GM, Der CJ, Wiley HS, Gill GN, Rosenfeld MG (1989) Functional independence of the epidermal growth factor receptor from a domain required for ligand-induced internalization and calcium regulation. Cell 59:33–43
15. Ciccodicola A, Dono R, Obici S, Simeone A, Zollo M, Perisco MG (1989) Molecular characterization of a gene of the EGF family expressed in undifferentiated human NTERA2 teratocarcinoma cells. EMBO 8:1987–1991
16. Coffey RJ, Derynck R, Wilcox JN, Bringman TS, Goustin AS, Moses HL, Pittelkow MR (1987) Production and auto-induction of transforming growth factor-α in human keratinocytes. Nature 328:817–820
17. Coleman S, Silberstein GG, Daniel CW (1988) Ductal morphogenesis in the mouse mammary gland: evidence supporting a role for epidermal growth factor. Dev Biol 127:304–315
18. Coleman S, Daniel CW (1990) Inhibition of mouse mammary ductal morphogenesis and down-regulation of the EGF receptor by epidermal growth factor. Dev Biol 137:425–433
19. Cook PW, Mattox P, Keeble A, Pittlekow WW, Plowman MR, Shoyab GD, Adelman JP, Shipley GD (1991) A heparin sulfate-regulated human keratinocyte autocrine factor is similar or identical to amphiregulin. Mol Cell Biol 11:2547–2557
20. Davis R, Like B, Massague J (1985) Modulation of type-α transforming growth factor receptors by a phorbol ester tumor promoter. J Cell Biochem 27:23–30
21. DeLarco JE, Todaro GJ (1978) Growth factors from murine sarcoma virus-transformed cells. Proc Natl Acad Sci USA 75:4001–4005
22. Derynck R (1988) Transforming growth factor α. Cell 54:593–595
23. Derynck R, Goeddel DV, Ullrich A, Gutterman JU, Williams RD, Brigman TS, Berger WH (1987) Synthesis of messenger RNAs for transforming growth factors α and β and the epidermal growth factor receptor by human tumors. Cancer Res 74:707–712
24. Derynck R, Roberts AB, Winkler ME, Chen EY, Goeddel DV (1984) Human transforming growth factor-α: precursor structure and expression in E. coli. Cell 38:287–297
25. Di Marco E, Pierce JH, Fleming TP, Kraus MH, Molloy CJ, Aaronson SA, DiFiore PP (1989) Autocrine interaction between TGFα and the EGF-receptor: quantitative requirements for induction of the malignant phenotype. Oncogene 4:831–838
26. DiFiore PP, Pierce JH, Fleming TP, Hazan R, Ullrich A, King CR, Schlessinger J, Aaronson SA (1987) Overexpression of the human EGF receptor confers an EGF-dependent transformed phenotype to NIH 3T3 cells. Cell 51:1063–1070
27. Farber E (1981) Chemical carcinogenesis. NEJM 305:1379–1389
28. Farber, E (1984) Precancerous steps in carcinogenesis: their physiological adaptive nature. Biochem Biophys Acta 738:171–180

29. Finzi E, Fleming T, Segatto O, Pennington CY, Bringman TS, Derynck R, Aaronson SA (1987) The human transforming growth factor type α coding sequence is not a direct-acting oncogene when overexpressed in NIH 3T3 cells. Proc Natl Acad Sci USA 84:3733–3737
30. Gain BS, Hollenberg MD, MacCannel KL, Lederis K, Winkler ME, Derynck R (1987) Distinct vascular actions of epidermal growth factor-urogastrone and transforming growth factor-α. J Pharmacol Exp Ther 242:331–337
31. Halter SA, Dempsey P, Matsui Y, Stokes MK, Graves-Deal R, Hogan BLM, Coffey RJ (1992) Distinctive patterns of hyperplasia in MMTV-TGFα transgenic mice: characterization of mammary gland and skin proliferations. Am J Path 140:1131–1146
32. Hendler FJ, Ozanne B (1984) Human squamous cell lung cancers express increased epidermal growth factor receptors. J Clin Invest 74:647–651
33. Higashiymama S, Abbraham JA, Miller J, Fiddes JC, Klagsburn M (1991) A heparin-binding growth factor secreted by macrophage-like cells that is related to EGF. Science 251:936–939
34. Holmes WE, Sliwkowski MX, Akita RW, Henzel WJ, Lee J, Park JW, Yansura D, Abadi N, Raab H, Lewis GD, Shepard MH (1992) Identification of heregulin, a specific activator of p185erbB2. Science 256:1205–1210
35. Inui T, Tusbura A, Morii S (1989) Incidence of precancerous foci of mammary glands and growth rate of transplantable mammary cancers in sialoadenctomized mice. J Natl Cancer Inst 81:1660–1663
36. Jhappan C, Stahle C, Harkins RN, Fausto N, Smith GH, Merlino GT (1990) TGFα overexpression in transgenic mice induces liver neoplasia and abnormal development of the mammary gland and pancreas. Cell 61:1137–1146
37. Ju WD, Velum TJ, Vass WC, Papageorge AG, Lowy DR (1991) Tumorigenic transformation of NIH 3T3 cells by the autocrine synthesis of transforming growth factor-α. New Biol 3:380–388
38. Kraus MH, Issing W, Miki T, Popescu NC, Aaronson SA (1989) Isolation and characterization of ERBB3, a third member of the ERBB/epidermal growth factor receptor family: evidence for overexpression in a subset of human mammary tumors. Proc Natl Acad Sci USA 86: 9193–9197
39. Kurachi H, Sokamoto, Oka T (1985) Evidence for the involvement of the submandibular gland epidermal growth factor in mouse mammary tumorigenesis. Proc Natl Acad Sci USA 82:5940–5943
40. Liu SC, Sanfilippo B, Perroteau I, Derynck R, Salomon DS, Kidwell WR (1987) Expression of transforming growth factor-α (TGF-α) in differentiated rat mammary tumors: estrogen induction of TGF-α production. Mol Endocrinol 1:683–692
41. Madtes DK, Raines EW, Sakariassen KS, Assoian RK, Sporn MB, Bell GI, Ross R (1988) Induction of transforming growth factor-α in activated human alveolar macrophages. Cell 53:285–295

42. Malden LT, Novak U, Burgess AW (1989) Expression of transforming growth factor alpha messenger RNA in the normal and neoplastic gastrointestinal tract. Int J Cancer 43:380–384

43. Markowitz SD, Molkentin K, Gerbic C, Jackson J, Stellato T, Wilson JKV (1990) Growth stimulation of coexpression of transforming growth factor-α and epidermal growth factor-receptor in normal and adenomatous human colon epithelium. J Clin Invest 86:356–362

44. Massague J (1990) Transforming growth factor-α: a model for membrane-anchored growth factors. J Biol Chem 265:21393–21396

45. Matsui Y, Halter SA, Holt JT, Hogan BLMR, Coffey RJ (1990) Development of mammary hyperplasia and neoplasia in MMTV-TGFα transgenic mice. Cell 61:1147–1155

46. McGeady ML, Kerby S, Shankar V, Ciardiello F, Salomon D, Seidman M (1989) Infection with a TGF-α retroviral vector transforms normal mouse mammary epithelial cells but not normal rat fibroblasts. Oncogene 4:1375–1382

47. Moolgavkar SH, Knudson AG (1981) Mutation and cancer. J Natl Cancer Inst 66:1037–1052

48. Moscat J, Molloy CJ, Fleming TP, Aaronson SA (1988) Epidermal growth factor activates phosphoinositide turnover and protein kinase C in BALB/MK keratinocytes. Mol Endocrinol 2:799–805

49. Opleta-Madsen K, Hardin J, Gall DG (1991) Epidermal growth factor up-regulates intestinal electrolyte and nutrient transport. Am J Physiol 260:G807–G814

50. Pandiella A, Massague J (1991) Cleavage of the membrane precursor for transforming growth factor-α is a regulated process. Proc Natl Acad Sci USA 88:1726–1730

51. Peles E, Bacus SS, Koski RA, Lu HS, Wen D, Ogden SG, Levy BR, Yarden Y (1992) Isolation of the New/HER-2 stimulatory ligand: a 44 kd glycoprotein that induces differentiation of mammary tumor cells. Cell 69:205–216

52. Pittelkow MR, Lindquist PB, Derynck R, Abraham RT, Graves-Deal R, Coffey RJ (1989) Induction of transforming growth factor-α expression in human keratinocytes by phorbol esters. J Biol Chem 264:5164–5171

53. Plowman GD, Green JM, McDonald VL, Neubauer MD, Disteche CM, Todaro GJ, Shoyab M (1990) The amphiregulin gene encodes a novel epidermal growth factor-related protein with tumor-inhibitory activity. Mol Cell Biol 10:169–1981

54. Roberts AB, Sporn MB (1990) The transforming growth factor-betas. In: Sporn MB, Roberts AB (eds) Peptide growth factors and their receptors I. Springer, Berlin Heidelberg New York, pp 419–472 (Handbook of experimental pharmacology, vol 95)

55. Rosenthal A, Lindquist PB, Bringman TS, Goeddel DV, Derynck D (1986) Expression in rat fibroblasts of a human transforming growth factor-α cDNA results in transformation. Cell 46:301–309

56. Sandgren EP, Luetteke NC, Palmiter RD, Brinster RL, Lee DC (1990) Overexpression of TGFα in transgenic mice: induction of epithelial hyperplasia, pancreatic metaplasia, and carcinoma of the breast. Cell 61:1121–1135

57. Schechter AL, Stern DF, Vaidyanathan L, Decker SJ, Drebin JA, Greene MI, Weinberg RA (1984) The neu oncogene: an erbB-related gene encoding a 185,000-Mr tumor antigen. Nature 312:513–516

58. Schreiber AB, Winkler ME, Derynck R (1986) Transforming growth factor-α: a more potent angiogenic mediator than epidermal growth factor. Science 232:1250–1253

59. Shankar V, Ciardiello F, Kim N, Derynck R, Liscia DS, Merlo G, Langton BC, Sheer D, Callahan R, Bassin RH, Lippman ME, Hynes N, Salomon DS (1989) Transformation of an established mouse mammary epithelial cell line following transfection with a human transforming growth factor alpha cDNA. Mol Carcin 2:1–11

60. Shoyab M, McDonald VL, Bradley JG, Todaro GJ (1988) Amphiregulin: a bifunctional growth-modulating glycoprotein produced by the phorbol 12-myristate 13-acetate-treated human breast adenocarcinoma cell line MCF-7. Proc Natl Acad Sci USA 85:6528–6532

61. Slamon DJ, Clark GM, Wong SG et al (1987) Human breast cancer: correlation of relapse and survival with amplification of the Her-2/neu oncogene. Science 235:177–182

62. Smith JA, Barraclough R, Fernig DG, Rudland PS (1989) Identification of alpha transforming growth factor as a possible local trophic agent for the mammary gland. J Cell Physiol 141:362–370

63. Snedeker SM, Brown CF, DiAgustine RP (1991) Expression and functional properties of transforming growth factor-α and epidermal growth factor during mouse mammary gland ductal morphogenesis. Proc Natl Acad Sci USA 88:276–280

64. Sporn MB, Todaro GJ (1980) Autocrine secretion and malignant transformation of cells. N Engl J Med 303:878–880

65. Thomas DM, Nasim MM, Gullick WJ, Alison MR (1992) Immunoreactivity of transforming growth factor alpha in the normal adult gastrointestinal tract. Gut 33:628–631

66. Todaro GJ, Fryling C, DeLarco JE (1980) Transforming growth factors produced by certain human tumor cells: polypeptides that interact with epidermal growth factor receptors. Proc Natl Acad Sci USA 77:5258–5262

67. Tonelli QJ, Sorof S (1980) Epidermal growth factor requirement for development of cultured mammary glands. Nature 285:250–252

68. Twardzik DR, Ranchalis JE, Todaro GJ (1982) Mouse embryonic transforming growth factors related to those isolated from tumor cells. Cancer Res 42:590–593

69. Vonderhaar BK (1984) Hormone and growth factors in mammary gland development. In: Veneziale CM (ed) Control of cell growth and proliferation. Van Nostrand-Reinhold, Princeton, pp 11–33

70. Vonderhaar BK (1987) Local effects of EGF, α-TGF, and EGF-like growth factors on lobuloalveolar development of the mouse mammary gland in vivo. J Cell Physiol 132:581–584
71. Wahl MI, Nishibe S, Kim S, Kim JW, Rhee SG, Carpenter G (1990) Identification of two epidermal growth factor-sensitive tyrosine phosphorylation sites of phospholipase C-g in intact HSC-1 cells. J Biol Chem 265:3944–3948
72. Wahl MI, Nishibe S, Suh PG, Rhee SG, Carpenter G (1989) Epidermal growth factor stimulates tyrosine phosphorylation of phospholipase C-II independently of receptor internalization and extracellular calcium. Proc Natl Acad Sci USA 86:1568–1572
73. Weinstein IB (1988) The origins of human cancer: molecular mechanisms of carcinogenesis and their implications for cancer prevention and treatment. Cancer Res 48:4135–4143
74. Wen D, Peles E, Cupples R, Suggs SV, Bacus SS, Luo Y, Trail G, Hu S, Silbiger SM, Levy BR, Koski RA, Lu HS, Yarden Y (1992) Neu differentiation factor: a transmembrane glycoprotein containing an EGF domain and an immunoglobulin homology unit. Cell 69:559–572
75. Wilcox JN, Derynck R (1988) Developmental expression of transforming growth factors alpha and beta in mouse fetus. Mol Cell Endocrinol 8:3415–3422
76. Wong ST, Winchell LF, McCune BK, Earp HS, Teixido J, Massague B, Herman DC, Lee DC (1989) The TGF-α precursor expressed on the cell surface binds to the EGF receptor on adjacent cells, leading to signal transduction. Cell 56:495–506
77. Wright NA, Pike C, Elia G (1990) Induction of a novel epidermal growth factor-secreting cell lineage by mucosal ulceration in human gastrointestinal stem cells. Nature 343:82–85
78. Yamamoto T, Kamata N, Kawano H, Shimizu S, Kuroki T, Toyoshima K, Rikimaru K, Nomura N, Ishizaki R, Pastan I, Gamon S, Shimizu N (1986) High incidence of amplification of the epidermal growth factor receptor gene in human squamous carcinoma cell lines. Cancer Res 46:414–416
79. Yuspa SH, Poirier MC (1988) Chemical carcinogenesis: from animal models to molecular models in one decade. Adv Cancer Res 50:25–70

7 Exploring the Pathogenic Potential of c-fos, Polyoma Middle T and Human Foamy Virus in Transgenic Mice

Erwin F. Wagner and Adriano Aguzzi

7.1 Introduction

The study of oncogenes represents a fascinating research area aimed at understanding their biochemical functions, their role in development, cellular proliferation and differentiation, and their causal involvement in diseases (Hanahan 1988; Weinberg 1989; Wagner 1990a,b). With regard to oncogenesis, numerous studies from different fields strongly imply a multistep model, suggesting that a series of events is required to convert a normal cell into an abnormally proliferating cell and, finally, into a malignant tumor cell. The dissection of the individual steps together with the identification of the genes responsible for the progression of a normal cell to a tumor cell is a major goal in current oncogene research. Whereas a large number of important studies on oncogene function are performed in cell culture systems, our focus lies in the elucidation of the role oncogenes play in mouse development and in the generation of mouse model systems to study human disease. We are using transgenic mice and embryonal stem (ES) cells as powerful systems to test the role of oncogenes in vivo (Wagner 1990 a,b; Robertson 1987) and we will also discuss our efforts to analyze the neuropathogenic potential of human foamy virus (HFV).

7.2 c-*fos* Expression in Transgenic and Chimeric Mice

To study the role of c-*fos* during development and to understand the specificity of *fos*-induced tumorigenesis we have made several DNA constructs in which the murine genomic c-*fos* gene was fused to different ubiquitous promoter elements in order to enable ectopic expression in a wide variety of tissues. Here, we will focus our discussion on the results obtained with transgenic mice harboring the H2-c-*fos*LTR construct, and chimeric mice harboring the MT-c-*fos*LTR construct. It should be noted that transgenic mice generated with using a MT-c-*fos*LTR construct develop a phenotype identical to the H2-c-*fos*LTR mice, but at a much lower penetrance (only 15%, see Rüther et al. 1987, 1989). Therefore, the latter family is more suitable for analysis of c-*fos* function and in regard to the ES cell experiments, only constructs with the hMT promoter have been used.

In H2-c-*fos*LTR transgenic mice, noticeable swellings were observed on the long bones as early as 4 weeks after birth, specifically in the areas of the distal femur and proximal tibia. These lesions increased significantly in size after only a few months and progressed to large calcified tumors in virtually all bones of the body (Fig. 1). The penetrance of osteosarcoma formation was 100 % as all mice carrying the transgene (that is, both heterozygotes and homozygotes) developed these tumors (Grigoriadis et al., submitted). The high penetrance and severity of the phenotype in H2-c-*fos*LTR mice enabled us to address specific questions on a background which was highly uniform.

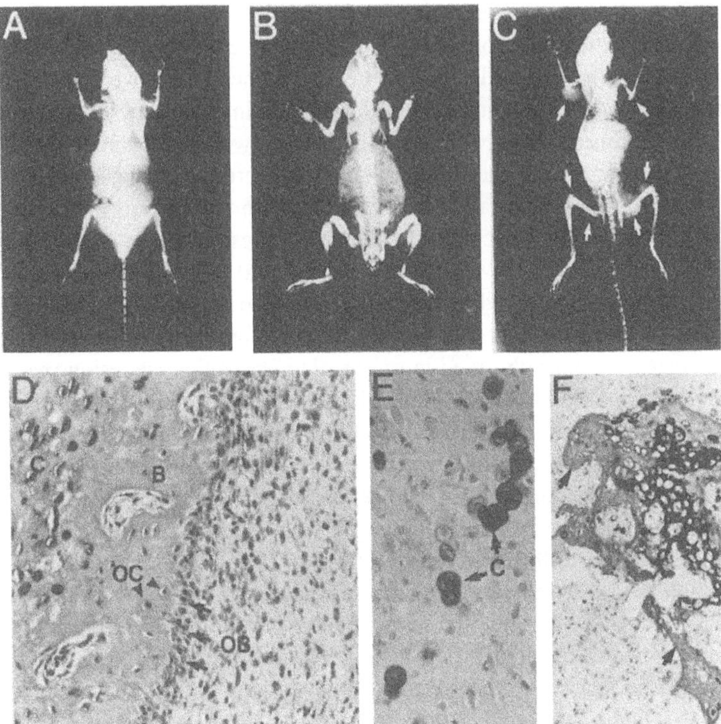

Fig. 1A–F. X-ray and histological analyses of the pathology observed in c-*fos* transgenic and chimeric mice. X-rays of a normal mouse (**A**), and H2-c-*fos*LTR transgenic mouse (**B**) and MT-c*fos*LTR chimeric mouse (**C**). Note the large calcified tumors present throughout the skeleton of the transgenic mouse compared to those present in the joints of the chimeric mouse (*arrows*). **D** A chondroblastic osteosarcoma from an H2-c-*fos*LTR transgenic mouse showing large areas of mineralized bone containing osteocytes (*OC, arrowheads*) and lined with cuboidal cells resembling osteoblasts (*OB, arrows*). In addition, areas of chondrocyte differentiation are also present. **E** Tumor from a MT-c-*fos*LTR chimeric mice showing a typical region containing chondrocytes (*c*) at different stages of differentiation. Some of the chimeric tumors contained areas of ossification surrounding the chondrocytes (*arrows* in **F**)

To address the consequences of ectopic c-*fos* expression during development, where endogenous levels show a very restricted pattern of expression, we isolated different ES cell clones which were selected for high c-*fos* expression and injected them into blastocysts. The resulting chimeric mice were all born healthy with no apparent abnormalities, suggesting that high levels of Fos protein during early embryonic development can be tolerated. However, as early as 3–4 weeks of age the chimeric mice developed palpable lesions in the areas of the spine and joints of the long bones (Wang et al. 1991), reminiscent of the phenotype observed in the transgenic mice. Upon further examination, however, it was evident that these lesions were different from the osteosarcomas observed in transgenic mice in that the lesions were generally not mineralized, although some contained sites of ossification (Fig. 1). Examination of the affected mice at autopsy confirmed the presence of large tumors associated with the spine, limbs, ribs and shoulders. The same phenotype was observed in chimeric mice generated from several different c-*fos*-expressing ES cell clones and the frequency of tumor formation ranged from 60 % to 100 %, depending on which *fos*-ES clone was used. These data suggest that the phenotype was not dependent upon the integration site of the DNA construct, but rather, was a result of c-*fos* overexpression during development. It should be mentioned that germline transmission has not yet been obtained, that is, we have not yet been able to show that the *fos*-ES cell derivatives have differentiated into functional germ cells. Thus, expression of exogenous c-*fos* in these chimeras can only occur in those tissues in which the *fos*-ES cells randomly contributed, and this contribution is different in each chimera. This is in contrast to the *fos* transgenic mice where all tissues in all animals contain the transgene, and each generation of mice develops the identical phenotype. Nevertheless, it is interesting that despite the random ES contribution in the *fos* chimeras, all mice develop the same phenotype (Wang et al. 1991).

Histological analysis was performed on both transgenic and chimeric tumors in order to characterize in greater detail the nature of the observed pathology. As shown in Fig. 1 the characteristics of each tumor are related but display fundamentally different properties. c-*fos* transgenic tumors resembled typical osteosarcomas, containing vast areas of osteoid and mineralized bone with cuboidal osteoblast-like cells lining areas of bone formation (Fig. 1D) and which also expressed high levels of alkaline phosphatase when stained histochemically. The tumors were vascularized and also contained areas of chondrocyte differentiation, which is typical of chondroblastic osteosarcomas (see also Rüther et al. 1989). In contrast, the hallmark of c-*fos* chimeric tumors was not bone formation but rather the presence of distinct foci of chondrogenic cells and differentiated chondrocytes surrounded by abundant extracellular matrix (Fig. 1E). The matrix stained intensely with Alcian blue and exhibited metachromasia after Toluidine blue staining, confirming the presence of sulfated proteoglycans which are abundant in cartilage matrix. Although the majority of tumors were unmineralized, a small number of tumors also contained areas of ossification (Fig. 1F). In transgenic osteosarcomas the tumors appeared to originate from regions corresponding to the periosteum of the long bones and consisted of areas of active bone formation. In contrast, the tumors in the *fos* chimeras were always associated with the joints and appeared to destroy the articular surfaces of the long bones. Since chondrocytes were the predominant cell type present in the *fos* chimera tumors, we have designated them as chondrogenic or chondrosarcoma-like tumors to distinguish them from the osteogenic and osteosarcoma-like tumors observed in the *fos* transgenic mice. In both cases, the tumors surrounded virtually the entire vertebral column and the long bones and were highly invasive as evidenced by the presence of ectopic bone and cartilage formation in the bone marrow spaces of transgenic and chimeric bones, respectively (data not shown). Thus, despite some similarities in skeletal localization, the tumors induced in the *fos* transgenic and chimeric mice are clearly different, suggesting that the affected cells in each tumor type may be different. Nevertheless, the cellular specificity of c-*fos* was reminiscent of the chondro-osseous neoplasms induced by the v-*fos*-containing FBJ- and FBR-MSVs (Ward and Young 1976).

To investigate exogenous c-*fos* expression in different transgenic and chimeric mouse tissues and to determine the tissue specificity of the transgene, we performed Northern blot analyses on tumor tissues as well as on unaffected tissues. In both transgenic and chimeric mice the highest levels of transgene expression were observed in the respective tumor tissues. In addition, stable expression of exogenous c-*fos* was detected in a wide variety of other tissues (Rüther et al. 1987; Wang et al. 1991; Grigoriadis et al., submitted), some at very high levels and in which no abnormalities were ever observed. Thus despite widespread and efficient expression in different tissues, the phenotypes generated were restricted to bone in the *fos* transgenics and to cartilage in the *fos* chimeras.

The complete penetrance of osteosarcoma formation in the transgenic mice enabled us to correlate the timing of exogenous c-*fos* expression with the onset of the phenotype, thereby addressing the causal role of c-*fos* in tumor formation. Time course experiments using Northern blot and X-ray analyses indicated that the transgene is first expressed in the bones of transgenic mice at approximately 2–3 weeks after birth, while the first evidence of pathological lesions was at 4 weeks of age (Grigoriadis et al., submitted). Therefore, expression of the transgene preceded the onset of the phenotype, implicating c-*fos* in the development of osteosarcomas in transgenic mice. With regard to chimeric mice, we have confirmed that exogenous Fos protein is expressed during embryogenesis, when the endogenous gene is normally not expressed. Specifically, expression was observed in several tissues of mesodermal and ectodermal origins, for example, in the developing prevertebral regions, thyroid gland, muscle and cervical ganglia (Wang et al. 1991). Taken together, the widespread tissue expression and the timing of expression suggest that high levels of c-*fos* can confer a specific growth advantage to osteogenic and chondrogenic cells.

Since all primary chondro- and osteosarcomas expressed high levels of exogenous c-*fos*, it was of interest to assess whether the expression of other genes was affected. To this end, we screened several tumors from different transgenic and chimeric mice for expression of AP-1-associated genes (e.g., endogenous c-*fos*, *fos*B, c-*jun*, *jun*B, *jun*D) and bone- and cartilage-associated genes (e.g., type I collagen, type II collagen, alkaline phosphatase, osteopontin, osteocalcin). These data demonstrate that primary transgenic osteosarcomas express high but variable levels of all osteoblast-associated markers tested, but not all AP-1 genes are expressed. One major difference between the osteogenic and chondrogenic tumors was in the expression of endogenous c-*fos*: Generally, the bone tumors did not express endogenous c-*fos* whereas the cartilage tumors coexpressed both endogenous and exogenous c-*fos* RNA. With respect to other AP-1 genes, it is of interest that c-*jun* levels in osteosarcomas were only moderately high while the chondrosarcomas expressed high levels of c-*jun* which appeared to correlate with the exogenous c-*fos* levels. In addition, the chondrosarcomas expressed the cartilage marker gene type II collagen, and interestingly, some bone markers as well.

7.2.1 Conclusion

In the above studies we have utilized two experimental systems to express high levels of exogenous Fos protein in mice. Both routes have enabled us to disrupt the normal physiological processes of mesenchymal cell development leading to specific tumors. The causal role of Fos in generating these phenotypes was demonstrated by several lines of evidence. First, exogenous c-*fos* was expressed in many different organs, yet only bone and cartilage tissues were affected, tissues which are also natural targets for the v-*fos* oncogene. Second, the timing of Fos expression indicated that it preceded the first morphological changes. In fact the observed time difference between expression of the transgene and appearance of early lesions in both transgenic and chimeric mice suggested that other events were required to elicit the observed biological effect. Third, the expression of the introduced gene in both transgenic and chimeric mice was highest in pathological tissues, specifically in different cell types, that is, in osteogenic cells in transgenic mice and chondrogenic cells in chimeric mice. Finally, and perhaps most importantly, cell lines isolated from each tumor type retained the ability to induce tumors in nude mice with similar morphological features to the original primary *fos*-induced tumors. Thus, osteosarcoma-derived cell lines gave rise to osteogenic tumors and cartilage tumor-derived cell lines induced cartilage tumors. Taken together, we have developed an experimental basis for postulating that there are two distinct but developmentally related target cell populations which are sensitive to high levels of Fos. Further experiments with mice lacking c-*fos* should substantiate the significance of these findings.

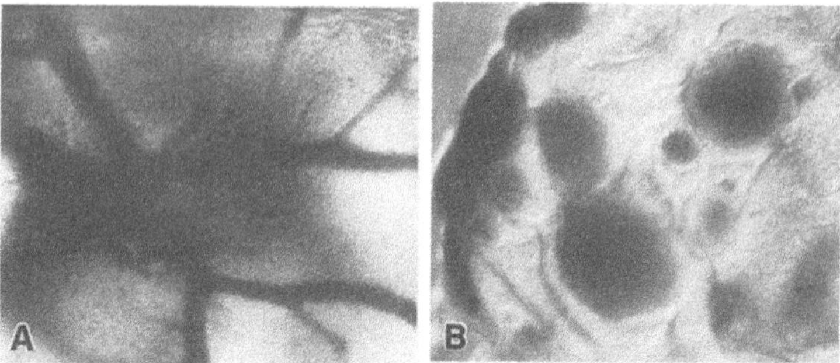

Fig. 2A,B. Disruption of the yolk sac vascular system in a Polyoma middle T (PymT) ES chimeric embryo at embrynic day E12.5. **A** Nonchimeric control. **B** Cavernous hemangiomas on yolk sac of PymT chimera

7.3 Polyoma Middle T Oncogene Expression and Vascular Tumors

The mT oncogene (PymT) was used to investigate whether a potent transforming gene that also influences the c-*src* kinase activity can exert dramatic effects on development when expressed in ES cells and early embryos. We generated an mT-carrying retrovirus and used it to infect ES cells. Individual clones were isolated that constitutively expressed mT and its associated tyrosine kinase activity. All chimeric embryos obtained by blastocyst injection of several ES cell clones died at midgestation when multiple hemangiomas disrupted blood vessel formation, particularly in the yolk sac (Fig. 2) (Williams et al. 1988). These experiments demonstrated that PymT specifically disrupts the growth control of endothelial cells, a finding supported by the fact that we were able to establish endothelioma (End) cell lines from chimeric embryos and from experimentally induced hemangiomas, as well as by direct infection of primary endothelial cells.

7.3.1 *PymT*, Endothelial Cells and Host Cell Recruitment

The End cell lines provided an excellent system for assessing the biological activity of mT, and we were astonished to see how rapidly (within 10–18 h after injection) they induced the formation of hemangiomas in various species, for example, mice, rats, chicks and quails (Williams et al. 1989; Aguzzi et al. 1991). A series of experiments using labeled End cells, in situ hybridization, and host cell-specific antibodies showed that over 95 % of the endothelial cells were host derived, thereby indicating that the intact End cells must act as a potent stimulating agent for the recruitment of nonproliferating host endothelial cells (Fig. 2) (Williams et al. 1989). The mechnism for this recruitment phenomenon is unclear.

7.3.2 *PymT*, Proteolytic Balance and Kinase Specificity

Our next experiments were aimed to study the morphogenetic properties of the End cells in an in vitro system. Using fibrin gels, we found that all End cell lines examined formed large hemangioma-like cystic structures and expressed high levels of fibrinolytic activity (Montesano et al. 1990). Increased production of urokinase-type plasminogen activator (u-PA) and reduced synthesis of PA inhibitors (PAI-1) were detected. The most astounding finding was that the neutralization of excess proteolytic activity by exogenously added serine protease inhibitors corrected the aberrant morphogenetic behavior and led to the formation of capillary-like tubules (Montesano et al. 1990). These results provide strong evidence that the mT oncogene modulates the expression of u-PA and, more significantly, of PAI-1 in endothelial cells, suggesting a causal relationship between the proteolytic activity and vascular morphogenesis. We have investigated a possible causal relationship between the high proteolytic activity displayed by End cells and their abnormal morphogenetic behavior using retroviral gene transfer of uPA and PAI-1. We found that expression of high levels of uPA following in vivo gene transfer into endothelia is compatible with normal angiogenesis. Presently, we aim to neutralize the excess proteolytic activity produced by End cells by overexpression of PAI-1 (F. Kiefer, unpublished data).

PymT has been shown to bind and activate the src family tyrosine kinases $pp60^{c\text{-}src}$, $p59^{fyn}$ and $pp62^{c\text{-}yes}$. In collaboration with P. Soriano we could demonstrate that hemangiomas are also efficiently formed in c-*src*-deficient mice following infection with PymT-transducing retrovirus (F. Kiefer, unpublished data). End cell lines derived from these lesions are indistinguishable from their src$^+$ counterparts. This implies that the association with pp60$^{c\text{-}src}$ is not necessary for the transformation of endothelial cells by PymT. Furthermore, the homologous mT oncogene of the hamster polyomavirus (HamT), which binds to pp59^{fyn} rather than to pp60$^{c\text{-}src}$, also causes hemangiomas in mice, however, at a significantly lower frequency and with longer latency period than mouse PymT (in collaboration with S. Courtneidge). Taken together, these data emphasize an important role of tyrosine kinases in the growth control of endothelial cells and of proteases and their inhibitors in angiogenesis and tissue repair.

7.4 Neuropathogenic Potential of Human Foamy Virus

While human retroviruses belonging to the oncoviral (human T-cell leukemia viruses, HTLV-I and -II) and lentiviral subgroup (human immunodeficiency viruses, HIV-I and II) have been extensively characterized as human pathogens, little is known about the pathogenic potential of HFV. This is surprising since the original identification of HFV precedes the discovery of HTLV and HIV by several years (Achong et al. 1971). HFV has been grouped together with bovine, simian and feline foamy viruses in a subfamily of retroviruses, spumaretrovirinae. The members of this subfamily share several structural properties, but are also related to some of the viruses classified as oncovirinae and lentivirinae (Mergia et al. 1990). The vacuolization observed in HFV-infected cultured cells led to its denomination as a "foamy" virus.

First isolated in a Kenyan patient suffering from nasopharyngeal carcinoma, HFV was subsequently found in patients suffering from diseases as diverse as de Quervain's thyroiditis (Stancek et al. 1975; Werner and Gelderblom 1979), encephalopathy (Cameron et al. 1978) and chronic myeloid leukemia (Young et al. 1973). Seroepidemiological studies showed that foamy virus infection is naturally prevalent in Pacific and East African populations where it reaches 3%–5% (Muller et al. 1980). African patients suffering from nasopharyngeal carcinoma and AIDS were found to have a much higher seroprevalence for HFV than healthy control individuals.

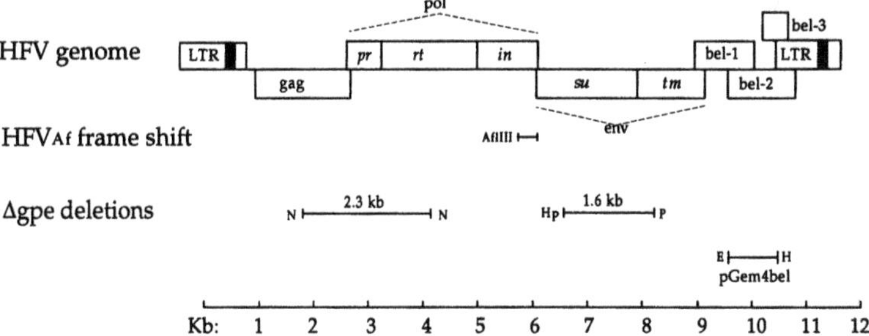

Fig. 3. Genomic organization of HFV and structure of the DNA fragments used to generate transgenic mice. In the *upper panel* the structure of wild-type HFV is depicted. In addition to *gag, pol* and *env*, HFV contains three ancillary reading frames designated *bel*-1 to *bel*-3. The *two lower panels* illustrate the structure of the constructs used for generation of transgenic mice. pHFV$_{Af}$ encodes the entire HFV genome rendered noninfectious by a frameshift mutation in its integrase domain, while pΔgpe contains two large deletions in the *gag-pol* and *env* genes, respectively. The *hatched areas* represent portions of the reading frames whose translation has been abrogated by the mutations

Despite these scattered clues to its pathogenicity it has never been convincingly demonstrated that HFV is the causative agent of any human disease and, indeed, HFV has often been considered a benign retrovirus. Similarly, simian, feline and bovine foamy viruses seem to induce persistent infections but have not yet been unequivocally associated with diseases despite their endemic character (Hooks and Detrick Hooks 1981). As a result, most of the interest in retroviral research has focused on oncoviruses and lentiviruses, which bear a definite and well-characterized pathogenic potential for their hosts, while the molecular and clinical analyses of foamy viruses have been somewhat neglected.

As shown in Fig. 3, the HFV genome is over 12 kb in length and, like all replication-competent retroviruses, encodes the structural genes gag (group specific antigen), pol (polymerase), and env (envelope). Although overall homology at the level of nucleotide sequence is not impressive, the detailed analysis of the genomic organization of HFV reveals striking similarities to the known human retroviruses, HTLV and HIV (Maurer et al. 1988). Of particular interest is the genomic region of HFV contained between the carboxyterminal portion of env and the 3'- long terminal repeat (LTR). Like the corresponding region in HTLV, this portion of the HFV genome has coding potential for at least three additional reading frames, which have been designated bel-1, bel-2 and bel-3 (the acronym bel signifies between env and LTR). Bel-1 encodes a transcriptional *trans*-acting factor essential for viral replication. The actual mechanism of transcriptional enhancement is still unclear, but it appears that bel-1 exerts its function indirectly and in an orientation-independent fashion. The function of the remaining reading frames is still unknown.

7.4.1 Studies of HFV Transgenic Mice

Since little information was available on the pathogenic properties of HFV in vivo, we have decided to explore the introduction of HFV genes into the germline of mice. The generation of transgenic mice has become a standard technique to investigate the consequences of expression of mammalian genes in whole organisms or in specific tissues (Wagner et al. 1990). In addition, transgenic mice have a distinct advantage over the use of infective virus in terms of biosafety, since introduction of appropriate mutations makes potentially hazardous spread of replication-competent viral particles highly unlikely. Two of the DNA constructs which have been introduced into fertilized mouse eggs are depicted in Fig. 3. The construct termed pHFVAf encodes the entire genome of HFV with a frameshift mutation in the endonuclease reading frame. This mutation disrupts a gene essential for proviral integration and ensures that infectious retroviral particles will not be assembled in cells expressing this construct.

In order to differentiate effects due to expression of the structural genes from those elicited by the ancillary bel genes, we have constructed an additional mutated form of HFV called pΔgpe, which contains two large deletions in the gag-pol and in the env regions of HFV (identified by horizontal bars in Fig. 3). The transcripts generated by this construct allow only for generation of truncated aminoterminal fragments of gag and env, while no pol gene products can be expressed. In contrast, the genes encoded by the bel genomic region are not affected by the introduced deletions and can be normally expressed. DNA analysis of tail tissue identified eight and nine pups containing pHFVAf and pΔgpe DNA, respectively. Several mice from the pΔgpe group passed the transgene to their progeny in a mendelian fashion, thus allowing establishment of transgenic lines.

Mice harboring either the pHFVAf or the pΔgpe construct developed a severe neurological syndrome at 6–8 weeks of age (Bothe et al. 1991; Aguzzi et al. 1992a). The most prominent neurological symptoms were ataxia and spastic tetraparesis. The symptoms rapidly progressed and led to death within 4–6 weeks from onset. The clinical features of this syndrome were similar in all animals, but transgenic mice harboring the pΔgpe construct displayed a later onset and slower progression than the mice expressing pHFVAf. With various morphological techniques we established that the pathological findings were restricted to the CNS and the striated muscles. By the age of 7 weeks most of the mice showed variable degrees of nerve cell loss in the forebrain, especially in the telencephalic cortex and in the CA3 layer of the hippocampus (Fig. 4). The lesions consisted of selective nerve cell degeneration with tissue atrophy and prominent reactive astrogliosis. At the borders between the lesions and the surrounding CNS tissue, degenerated nerve cells were present with condensed, highly eosinophilic cytoplasm. In addition, two founder animals and all their progeny were found to develop by the age of 2 months a total degeneration of the cerebellar granule cell layer in addition to the findings described. Clinically, these mice suffered from an obvious cerebellar phenotype, consisting mainly of ataxia (C. Kretschmer, K. Bothe, and A. Aguzzi, unpublished observations). Several mice analyzed exhibited foci of degeneration in the striated muscles ranging from atrophy of single myotubes to large areas with extensive necroses.

In addition to the neuro- and myodegenerative disease described above, further pathological changes were seen in transgenic founder mice carrying the pHFVAf construct. Macroscopic examination of the brain in these mice revealed a peculiar appearance of the cerebellar white matter with spotty symmetric areas of grayish color, suggestive of plaques of demyelination. Histopathological analysis confirmed severe bilateral damage of the myelinated tracts in forebrain, brain stem, cerebellum, and in a milder form, in the spinal cord. The most dramatic phenotype was observed in the anterior commissure and the corpus callosum, the optic nerves and the optic chiasm, and the cere-

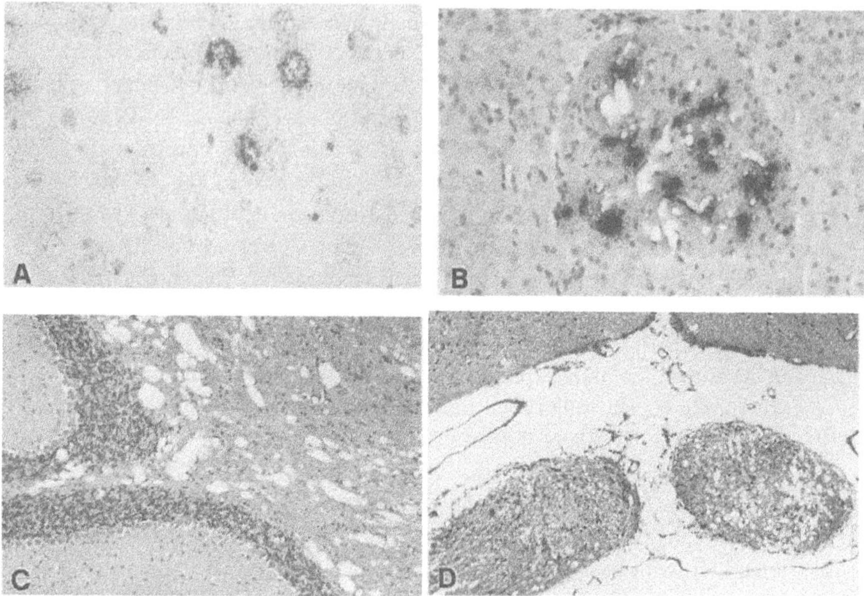

Fig. 4A–D. Pathology induced by human foamy virus (HFV) in transgenic mice

bellar white matter. These lesions were invariably associated with numerous non-neuronal cells expressing the HFV transgene. The microscopic appearance of these white matter lesions revealed a spongy myelinopathy with microcystic changes of variable diameter. However, areas of true demyelination were not present and the staining intensity of myelin between the vacuoles was roughly normal. Bodian stains and electron microscopic studies of selected animals did not disclose evidence of a primary axonal lesion, but immunocytochemistry for glial fibrillary acidic protein (GFAP) revealed pronounced astrogliosis. These additional pathologies in the white matter led to more severe symptoms than the phenotype observed in pΔgpe transgenic mice and suggest that expression of yet unidentified components of the structural genes may be specifically toxic to the myelination system.

7.4.2 Developmental Expression of HFV in Transgenic Mice

In order to gain a better understanding of the relationship between expression of HFV and the development of the disease, we have studied the time course of expression of the HFV transgene during development using in situ hybridization (Aguzzi et al. 1992b). We found that HFV was widely expressed at low levels and well tolerated during development, and that its pattern of expression differed from that of known retroviruses. Transcription of HFV occurred in two distinct phases. At midgestation, widespread expression was first detected in cells of the extra-embryonic membranes and in various tissues originating from mesoderm, neuroectoderm and neural crest. Expression decreased dramatically during late gestation. Surprisingly, the highest levels of expression achieved during embryonic life were not found in the neural tube, but in neural crest-derived tissues, such as the dorsal root ganglia. No permanent morphological damage was detected during this time and expression was suppressed in most tissues shortly after birth. However, several weeks later transcription of HFV resumed in a small fraction of single cells distributed irregularly in the central nervous system and in the skeletal muscle. At the age of 6–8 weeks expression reached extremely high levels in an increasing number of cells in these tissues and was followed by severe degenerative changes. These findings indicate that the regulatory elements of HFV allow for expression in a broad range of tissues at midgestation and that tissue-specific expression of HFV is differentially regulated later in development. Detailed molecular analysis of the events responsible for these observations may shed light on the mechanisms controlling retroviral latency and perhaps also on some aspects of vertical transmission of retroviruses.

7.4.3 Mechanisms of Neurotoxicity

The developmental profile of HFV gene expression in transgenic mice suggests that cytotoxicity is achieved only when a threshold expression is reached, and low levels of transcription, such as those observed during prenatal life, seem to be tolerated. However, the actual mechanism by which HFV induces tissue degeneration in the CNS and striated muscle is still unclear. The most basic question with respect to pathogenesis is: which of the HFV genes are cytotoxic? At present we are speculating that bel-1 represents a likely candidate for neurotoxicity. This would be in agreement with the neurotoxic properties of functionally analogous lentiviral transactivators such as the tat molecules of HIV and visna-maedi virus. In addition, we have not been able to overexpress high levels of bel-1 in fibroblastic cell lines, whereas subliminal levels of expression are tolerated (A. Aguzzi and E. F. Wagner, unpublished data). This suggests that high concentrations of bel-1 may be generally cytotoxic. Bel-1 may exert transactivating functions on cellular genes in addition to the LTR of HFV, and resulting perturbations of gene expression may play a role in neurotoxicity. In addition, the spotty distribution of cells expressing bel genes observed in in situ hybridization studies suggests that bel-1 is capable of initiating a positive feedback loop of retroviral transactivation to single cells. This may lead to extremely high levels of transcriptional activity and to cytopathic effects.

Notwithstanding this circumstantial evidence, we cannot exclude that the aminoterminal portions of gag and/or env contribute to the phenotype observed. Truncated forms of these gene products may be translated from the microinjected constructs and play a role in at least a part of the spectrum of diseases observed.

7.4.4 Conclusions

The HFV transgenic mice discussed in the present article represent a novel development in human retrovirology, since this model system has provided the first clear-cut evidence of pathogenicity of HFV. However, caution has to be exercised when trying to draw from a transgenic animal model conclusions valid for the natural route of infection, since the transgenic biology may differ in many important aspects from horizontal spread of infective retroviral particles. In particular, all somatic and germ cells of a transgenic mouse contain the transgenic DNA in equal amounts, in contrast to horizontal transmission through the natural route. Despite this limitation, the transgenic mouse model has enabled us to address questions not easily accessible by other means. Further, deletion of portions of the genome may create replication-defective mutants and mimic abortive retroviral infection, which seems to play a role in some forms of neuronal degeneration (Sharpe et al. 1990). Finally, we have shown that in the case of the HFV mice expression could be achieved in early embryonic stages, thus simulating some aspects of transplacental infection.

The neurodegenerative and myopathic pathologies induced by HFV in transgenic mice forces us to reevaluate the potential dangers of HFV infection for humans, particularly in view of the high prevalence of HFV in specific geographic areas. HFV was once found in the brain of a patient suffering from a neurodegenerative disease (Cameron et al. 1978), and the description of the neuropathology of the patient's brain was intriguingly reminiscent of the lesions developing in the HFV mice.

Certain intriguing similarities of the phenotype of HFV transgenic mice to known human retroviral diseases prompt us to extend our speculations on the possible role of HFV in human medicine. Other human retroviruses, such as HTLV-I and HIV, are frequently associated with neurological syndromes. While HTLV-I infection often results in spinal motor neuron degeneration, a majority of AIDS patients develop complex and variable pathologies of the CNS during their illness (Petito 1988; Gonzales and Davis 1988). CNS involvement in adult AIDS patients is most often characterized by a microglial nodular encephalitis, opportunistic infections, and a progressive diffuse encephalopathy of the white matter (Kleihues et al. 1985). While these features were not observed in HFV mice, AIDS encephalopathy following congenital and early childhood HIV infection often presents with distinct features, including nerve cell loss and subcortical necroses (Giangaspero et al. 1989; Lewis et al. 1990), which are reminiscent of the neuropathological changes in HFV mice.

In addition, the microcystic changes seen in the pHFVAf mice resemble a condition called vacuolar myelopathy, which occurs in the spinal cord of 10 %–20 % of AIDS patients (Petito et al. 1985; Maier et al. 1989). Vacuolar myelopathy affects the myelin sheaths of the long tracts of the cord while sparing the axons, and closely resembles subacute combined degeneration. As in HFV myelinopathy, vacuolar myelopathy often occurs in the absence of a significant cellular reaction and is probably due to a direct toxic action of retroviral gene products. The morphological analogies between the HFV phenotype and this condition, together with the reported difficulties to isolate HIV from vacuolar myelopathic lesions, suggests that it will be important to search for coinfection with HFV in AIDS patients developing spinal cord pathologies.

References

Achong BG, Mansell PW, Epstein MA, Clifford P (1971) An unusual virus in cultures from a human nasopharyngeal carcinoma. J Natl Cancer Inst 46: 299–307

Aguzzi A, Kleihues P, Heckl K, and Wiestler OD (1991) Cell type specific tumor induction by oncogens in fetal forebrains transplants. Oncogene 6:113–118

Aguzzi A, Bothe K, Wagner EF, Rethwilm A, Horak I (1992a) Human Foamy Virus: an underestimated neuropathogen? Brain Pathol 2:61–69

Aguzzi A, Bothe K, Horak I, Rethwilm A, Anhauser I, Wagner EF (1992b) Developmental modulation of human foamy virus expression. The New Biologist 4:225–237

Bothe K, Aguzzi A, Lassmann H, Rethwilm A, Horak I (1991) Progressive encephalopathy and myopathy in transgenic mice expressing human foamy virus genes. Science 253:555–557

Cameron KR, Birchall SM, Moses MA (1978) Isolation of foamy virus from patient with dialysis encephalopathy. Lancet 2:79666

Giangaspero F, Scanabissi E, Baldacci MC, Betts CM (1989) Massive neuronal destruction in human immunodeficiency virus (HIV) encephalitis. A clinico-pathological study of a pediatric case. Acta Neuropathol Berl 78:662–665

Gonzales MF, Davis RL (1988) Neuropathology of acquired immunodeficiency syndrome. Neuropathol Appl Neurobiol 14:345–363

Hanahan D (1988) Dissecting multistep tumorigenesis in transgenic mice. Annu. Rev. Genet. 22:479–519

Hooks JJ, Detrick-Hooks B (1981) In: Kurstak E, Kurstak C (eds) Comparative diagnosis of viral diseases. Academic Press: New York, pp 599–618

Kleihues P, Lang W, Burger PC, Budka H, Vogt M, Maurer R, Lüthy R, Siegenthaler W (1985) Progressive diffuse leukoencephalopathy in patients with acquired immunodeficiency syndrome (AIDS). Acta Neuropathol Berl 333:339

Lewis SH, Reynolds-Kohler C, Fox HE, Nelson JA (1990) HIV-1 in trophoblastic and villous Hofbauer cells, and haematological precursors in eight-week fetuses. Lancet 335: 565–568

Maier H, Budka H, Lassmann H, Pohl P (1989) Vacuolar myelopathy with multinucleated giant cells in the acquired immune deficiency syndrome (AIDS). Light and electron microscopic distribution of human immuno-deficiency virus (HIV) antigens. Acta Neuropathol Berl 78:497–503

Maurer B, Bannert H, Darai G, Flügel RM (1988) Analysis of the primary structure of the long terminal repeat and the gag and pol genes of the human spumaretrovirus. J Virol 62:1590–1597

Mergia A, Shaw KE, Lackner JE, Luciw PA (1990) Relationship of the env genes and the endonuclease domain of the pol genes of simian foamy virus type 1 and human foamy virus. J Virol 64:406–410

Montesano R, Pepper MS, Möhle-Steinlen U, Rissau W, Wagner EF, Orci L (1990) Increased proteolytic activity is responsible for the aberrant morphogenetic behavior of endothelial cells expressing middle T oncogene. Cell 62:435–445

Muller HK, Ball G, Epstein MA, Achong BG, Lenoir G, Levin A (1980) The prevalence of naturally occurring antibodies to human syncytial virus in East African populations. J Gen Virol 47:399–406

Petito CK (1988) Review of central nervous system pathology in human immunodeficiency virus infection. Ann Neurol 23 Suppl: S54–S57

Petito CK, Navia BA, Cho ES, Jordan BD, George DC, Price RW (1985) Vacuolar myelopathy pathologically resembling subacute combined degeneration in patients with the acquired immunodeficiency syndrome. N Engl J Med 312:874–879

Robertson EJ (1987) In: Teratocarcinomas and embryonic stem cells: A practical approach. IRL Press, Oxford

Rüther U, Garber C, Komitowski D, Müller R and Wagner EF (1987) Deregulated c-*fos* expression interferes with normal bone development in transgenic mice. Nature 325:412–416

Rüther U, Komitowski D, Schubert FR, Wagner EF (1989) c-*fos* expression induces bone tumors in transgenic mice. Oncogene 4:861–865

Sharpe AH, Hunter JJ, Chassler P, Jänisch R (1990) Role of abortive retroviral infection of neurons in spongiform CNS degeneration. Nature 346: 181–183

Stancek D, Stancekova-Gressnerova M, Janotka M, Hnilica P, Oravec D (1975) Isolation and some serological and epidemiological data on the viruses recovered from patients with subacute thyroiditis de Quervain. Med Microbiol Immunol Berl 161:133–144

Wagner EF (1990a) Oncogenes and transgenic mice. In: Habenicht A (ed) Growth factors, differentiation factors and cytokines, Springer-Verlag, Berlin, pp 366–380

Wagner EF (1990b) On transferring genes into stem cells and mice (EMBO medal Review) EMBO J 9:3025–3032

Wang ZQ, Grigoriadis AE, Möhle-Steinlein U, Wagner EF (1991) A novel target cell for c-*fos*-induced oncogenesis: Development of chondorgenic tumors in embryonic stem cell chimaeras. EMBO J 10:2437–2350

Ward JM, Young D (1976) Histogenesis and morphology of periosteal sarcomas induced by FBJ virus in NIH Swiss mice. Cancer Res. 36: 3985–3992

Weinberg RA (1989) In: Oncogenes and molecular origins of Cancer, Cold Spring Harbor Laboratory Press, Cold Spring Harbor, New York

Werner J, Gelderblom H (1979) Isolation of foamy virus from patients with de Quervain thyroiditis. Lancet 2:258–259

Williams RL, Courtneidge SA, Wagner EF (1988) Embryonic lethalities and endothelial tumors in chimaeric mice expressing polyoma virus middle T oncogene. Cell 52:121–131

Williams RL, Risau W, Zerwes HG, Drexler H, Aguzzi A, and Wagner EF (1989) Endothelioma cells expressing the polyoma middle T oncogene induce hemangiomas by host cell recruitment. Cell 57:1053–1063

Young D, Samuels J, Clarke JK (1973) A foamy virus of possible human origin isolated in BHK-21 cells. Arch Gesamte Virusforsch 42:228–234

8 Transgenic Animals as Bioreactors for Therapeutic and Nutritional Proteins

Lothar Hennighausen, Avi Shamay, Priscilla A. Furth,
Robert A. McKnight, Caird Rexroad Jr, Vern G. Pursel,
and Robert J. Wall

8.1 Introduction: Accomplishments

The development of molecular "pharming" technology culminated in transgenic animals whose mammary glands were converted into bioreactors producing human proteins. This was achieved with interdigitative efforts by several branches of science — molecular biology, embryology, and protein chemistry. Protein chemistry helps to identify sequences of milk proteins, molecular biology provides the tools for the isolation of genetic regulatory elements that target gene expression to mammary tissue, and embryology is critical for the introduction of novel genes into embryos from which transgenic animals are derived. An important focus of current investigation in the field of mammary biotechnology comes from our accumulating understanding of molecular gene switches in the context of complex chromatin.

Pioneering work in the 1970s by Mercier and coworkers provided the amino acid sequences of several milk proteins. From this information, the cDNAs of several milk proteins were rapidly cloned and sequenced in the early 1980s using the then emerging cloning technologies (Hobbs et al. 1982; Hennighausen and Sippel 1982b). This provided the DNA sequences for known caseins and whey proteins and, in additon, resulted in the identification of novel proteins, such as the whey acidic protein (WAP) (Hennighausen and Sippel 1982a). Using milk protein cDNAs as probes, genomic clones for WAP, α-lactalbumin and several caseins were isolated and extensively characterized using in vitro systems (for review see Hennighausen 1992). Transgenic technologies established in the early 1980s resulted in the introduction of a foreign gene into the germline of transgenic animals, modifying the physiology of the organism (Palmiter et al. 1982). However, it was not until 1987 that researchers showed that regulatory elements from the mouse WAP gene could direct production of human proteins in mammary tissue of transgenic animals. Groner and coworkers successfully produced the human ras protein in mammary tissue (Andres et al. 1987). A joint research venture between Heiner Westphal's group and our laboratory at the National Institutes of Health in Bethesda and Katie Gordon at Integrated Genetics in Framingham demonstrated that lactating transgenic mice could secrete active human tissue plasminogen activator (tPA) into their milk (Gordon et al. 1987). In the same year researchers at the AFRC in Edinburgh demonstrated that mammary regulatory elements could function across species boundaries (Simons et al. 1987). The same group showed the feasibility of producing human proteins in sheep milk, although expression levels obtained were very low (Clark et al. 1989). In 1991, collaborative research between the NIH and the USDA demonstrated that gram quantities of a foreign protein could be produced in transgenic swine (Wall et al. 1991). Researchers from Pharmaceutical Proteins Limited and the AFRC in Edinburgh generated transgenic sheep that produced gram quantities of human α1-antitrypsin in their milk (Wright et al. 1991). Scientists from Tufts University and Genzyme showed production of human tPA in goat milk (Ebert et al. 1991; Denman et al. 1991), while work from Genpharming in Leiden resulted in transgenic cows carrying a human lactoferrin gene under the control of a casein promoter (Krimpenfort et al. 1991). Although this work represented major progress, one note of caution was also reported. Aberrant expression of a foreign protein in milk could interfere with mammary development and abrogate mammary function, resulting in

milchlos phenotypes (Burdon et al. 1991b; Shamay et al. 1992b). Finally, gene transfer systems have been developed which allow the introduction of DNA into mammary epithelium of pregnant and lactating animals in vivo (Furth et al. 1992) and in vitro (Furth et al. 1992; Yang et al. 1990). Such systems may permit a rapid evaluation of hybrid genes in the context of the farm animal of choice.

8.2 Milk Protein Genes
and the Mammary Gland Bioreactor

8.2.1 Rationales for Mammary Bioreactors

Although it is possible to produce human proteins on a large scale in manipulated microorganisms, there are limitations to these systems since many proteins require extensive post-translational modification. Factor IX is a good example in that this essential component for blood coagulation is normally synthesized in liver and undergoes extensive post-translational modifications that include glycosylation, β-hydroxylation and vitamin K-dependent γ-carboxylation (Di Scipio et al. 1978). In contrast to microorganisms, mammalian tissue culture cells contain the enzymatic machinery for these types of modifications of proteins. Since it is both technically challenging and expensive to grow many cell types in tissue culture on a large enough scale to produce high yields of protein, current efforts are being directed toward alternative measures. One such system may be the mammary gland bioreactor. During lactation the mammary gland synthesizes large amounts of protein which is secreted into the milk in concentrations between 40 and 60 g/l. By targeting the expression of foreign genes to the mammary gland in transgenic animals it may be possible to produce human proteins on this scale in milk. This translates to about 20 kg or 100 kg for a goat or cow, respectively, per year. Although the expense of generating transgenic livestock are high, husbandry is relatively cheap and only low-tech facilities are needed. These assets of transgenic technology can be contrasted to expensive fermenters for cells in culture and the cost of growth media for fastidious cell lines.

In addition to high value human pharmaceuticals, the mammary bioreactor can be used to produce food additives such as human lactoferrin to supplement infant formula. Other long-term goals are the generation of cows with an increased casein content in milk.

8.2.2 Milk Protein Genes

A plethora of milk protein genes from several species have been isolated (for review see Hennighausen 1992). These include α-lactalbumin genes from rat, human, bovine, guinea pig and caprine, WAP genes from mice, rats and rabbits, the β-lactoglobulin gene from sheep, β-casein genes from mice, rats, bovine and goats, and α-casein genes from rat, and bovine. Using transgenic technology mammary specificity has been attributed to promoter upstream sequences in the WAP, β-lactoglobulin, α-casein, β-casein and α-lactalbumin genes. However, in the context of the whole organism no single mammary regulatory element has been identified yet. Although many milk proteins are shared between species, some proteins are unique to the milk of certain species. WAP, for example, has only been found in mice, rats, rabbits and camels, and β-lactoglobulin is absent from mice, rats and camels. However, mammary regulatory elements have been conserved during evolution and between different species. This is exemplified with the mouse WAP gene which is well expressed in transgenic pigs (Wall et al. 1991) and sheep (Fig. 1). Transgenic pigs and sheep were generated carrying a 7-kb fragment containing the mouse WAP gene including promoter/upstream and 3'-flanking sequences and the encoded RNA was only found in mammary tissue (Fig. 1) and the protein was accurately translated (unpublished).

Developmental and hormonal regulation between milk protein genes varies significantly (Hobbs et al. 1982). For example, accumulation of WAP (Pittius et al. 1988) RNA occurs just prior to parturition, but high levels of β-casein mRNA are detected in early pregnancy (Harris et al. 1991; Hennighausen et al. 1988; Shamay et al. 1992a). Differences in regulation may be the result of differential access of

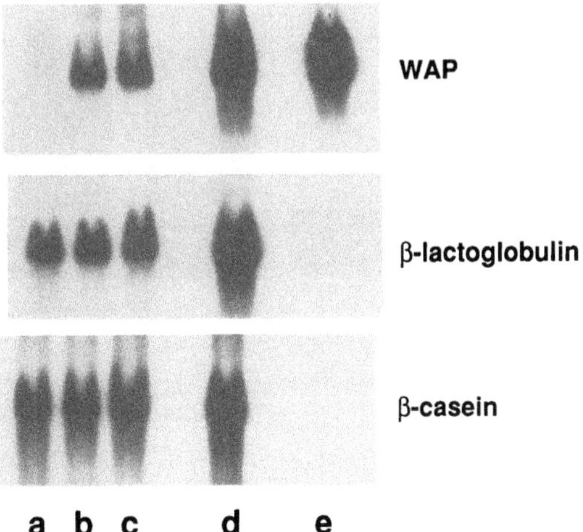

Fig. 1. Expression of mouse WAP transgenes in sheep. Mammary RNA from a lactating nontransgenic ewe (*lane a*), from two transgenic founder ewes (ewe 029 in *lane b* and ewe 001 in *lane c*), from a lactating pig carrying the mouse WAP transgene (*lane d*; Wall et al. 1991) and from a lactating nontransgenic mouse (*lane e*) was separated in a 1.5 % formaldehyde gel, blotted onto a nylon membrane, and successively hybridized with a mouse WAP cDNA, a swine β-lactoglobulin and a swine β-casein probe

chromatin to individual signaling pathways. Evidence for this comes from transgenic studies with the WAP gene in transgenic mice (Burdon et al. 1991a,b; Pittius et al. 1988) and pigs (Shamay et al. 1992a). Developmental and hormonal induction patterns obtained with WAP transgenes varied substantially with the integration site (Shamay et al. 1992a) and critical chromatin components, such as matrix attachment regions (MAR) may be necessary for accurate regulation (McKnight et al. 1992).

8.2.3 From Mice to Farm Animals

Transgenic mice which secrete human pharmaceuticals into milk have been established as model systems (Hennighausen 1990). However,

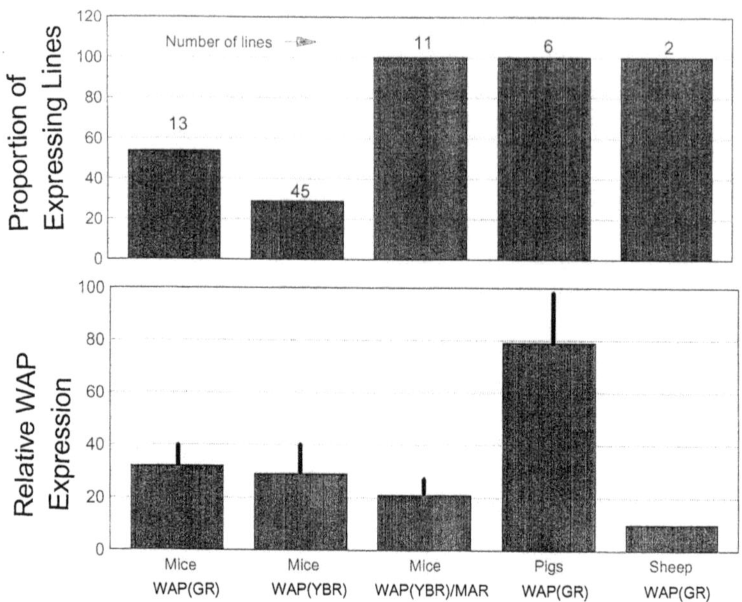

Fig. 2. Compiled data of WAP transgene expression in mice, pigs and sheep. The proportion of expressing lines of transgenic animals is shown in the *upper panel*, and the relative expression levels in the *lower panel*. A total of 13 lines of transgenic mice carrying a WAP gene from the GR strain (Burdon et al. 1991), 45 mouse lines carrying the WAP gene from the YBR strain, 11 mouse lines carrying the WAP gene from the YBR strain and MAR sequences (McKnight et al. 1992), six lines of transgenic pigs (Wall et al. 1991) and two lines of transgenic sheep

the conclusions obtained with these model systems may not necessarily be transferable to farm animals. This notion is strongly supported by extensive studies that have been conducted with the mouse WAP gene in transgenic mice, pigs and sheep which do not contain a recognizable endogenous WAP gene. The mouse WAP transgene was expressed in a tight mammary specific fashion in all three species, suggesting that the molecular basis of mammary-specific gene expression is conserved between species and probably between different milk protein genes (Fig. 2). Surprisingly, the frequency of expressors and expression levels between these species varied sharply (Fig. 2). While only about 50 % of the mice express the WAP transgene, it was expressed at high levels in all transgenic pigs and sheep. Similarly, expression levels of a hybrid gene containing WAP regulatory elements and human protein C sequences were dramatically higher in pigs than in mice (Velander et al. 1992). Finally, a sheep β-lactoglobulin gene was expressed at high levels in transgenic mice (Simons et al. 1987) which also do not contain an endogenous counterpart. It may well turn out that expression levels are higher upon crossing species boundaries.

8.2.4 Designer Genes

Promoter/upstream sequences from the WAP, α-casein, α-lactalbumin, β-lactoglobulin, and the β-casein gene have been used to direct the synthesis of foreign proteins to mammary tissue of transgenic mice, rabbits, sheep and pigs (for references see Wilmut et al. 1991; Ebert et al. 1991; Wright et al. 1991; Hennighausen 1990, 1992). In general, genomic clones appear to be expressed at higher levels than cDNAs. Whereas expression of cDNA sequences encoding non-milk proteins under the control of milk protein gene-specific regulatory elements has been overall poor, genomic sequences linked to milk protein promoter elements showed greatly improved expression levels (Archibald et al., 1990). Increased activity of intron-containing transgenes may be the result of splicing (Brinster et al. 1988; Palmiter et al. 1991; Choi et al. 1991) or to the presence of regulatory elements located in specific introns. The particular reporter gene used can also influence expression levels and expression of recombinant genes can greatly vary between different species.

In many cases transgenes are not expressed because they are subject to position effects imposed by the site of integration. MARs are sequences which help to functionally separate genes from surrounding chromatin/regulatory regions, possibly by anchoring genetic domains to the nuclear matrix (Bonifer et al. 1991). When WAP transgenes were coinjected with MAR elements, accurate expression was found in almost all lines, suggesting that such "insulator" sequences may be helpful in obtaining more expressing transgenic lines for any given transgene (McKnight et al. 1991). Since DNA fragments coinjected into fertilized oocytes will in many cases integrate into the same transgene locus (Burdon et al. 1991a; Overbeek et al. 1991; McKnight et al. 1992), this strategy should allow the generation of transgenic animals that carry several different hybrid genes and therefore secrete several different proteins into their milk.

8.3 The Next Decade

Three developments may increase the pace of introducing mammary bioreactors on a large scale into the industrial complex. The isolation of elements that build genetic chromatin domains, in vivo gene transfer systems to be used as screening systems to rapidly evaluate hybrid genes, and the development of embryonic stem cells.

In general, animals from about 50% of transgenic lines express a given transgene, and expression is highly variable and position dependent. Moreover, expression levels between animals from a defined genetic line may vary considerably. Recent technological advances allow shielding of transgenes from integration site-dependent position effects. This should permit the reproducible establishment of transgenic lines which produce a given protein at similar high levels. MARs and locus control regions (LCRs) are experimental systems which may aid our efforts to consistently express transgenes at high levels. MARs appear to define genetic units, and their presence prevents "spill-over" of regulatory signals between neighboring genetic domains (Bonifer et al. 1991). Without MAR sequences, expression and regulation of mammary-directed transgenes is highly position dependent, whereas accurate regulation was obtained in the presence of heterologous MARs from the chicken lysozyme locus (McKnight et al. 1992). In contrast to MARs, whose sole function appears to be to shield genetic domains, LCR are *cis*-acting elements which probably contain enhancers that confer position-independent expression to genes in transgenic loci (Grosveld et al. 1987). The utilization of MAR- and/or LCR-like sequences may be necessary to reach the biotechnological goal. It may not be necessary to build such elements into expression vectors, because the coinjection of MARs with hybrid genes normally results in cointegration in the same transgenic locus (McKnight et al. 1992). From a pragmatic point of view, significant benefits may be realized by including either homologous or heterologous MARs with transgene constructs in transgenic livestock. The proportion of transgenic large animals that express their transgene is approximately 60%. Given that the cost of producing transgenic sheep and pigs is in the tens of thousands of dollars, and production of transgenic cattle may be an order of magnitude higher, the use of MARs could substantially reduce transgenic animal production costs.

The inclusion of MAR sequences in a transgenic locus may also result in accurate transgene regulation (McKnight et al. 1992) which may be of particular importance in the light of potential cytotoxic effects caused by some proteins. For example, precocious expression of WAP in both transgenic mice (Burdon et al. 1991b) and swine (Shamay et al. 1992b) resulted in impaired mammary development during pregnancy and a *milchlos* phenotype.

Most mammary transgenes analyzed to date yielded suboptimal expression levels, suggesting that critical elements involved in transcription, RNA processing, or mRNA stabilization were missing from the hybrid gene. In addition, de novo combination of sequences in hybrid gene may interfere with optimal regulation. Since the evaluation of hybrid genes in transgenic mice is time consuming, expensive, and the results may not always apply to farm animals, it is necessary to devise fast and reliable assay systems. The physical introduction of DNA via jet injection into mammary epithelial cells of living animals presents such a screening method (Furth et al. 1992). This permits the analysis of mammary vector systems in the context of the dairy animal which has also been chosen for the production of any particular protein. This technology should also permit the introduction of DNA into mammary epithelial stem cells to generate somatic transgenic cows. Bypassing the germline would cut the lead time by several years. Alternatively, DNA can be introduced in vitro into mammary tissue using the gold particle bombardment technique (Yang et al. 1990).

Although transgenic animals have permitted the development of the mammary bioreactor, this technology is limited in that the sites of transgene integration into the genome appear to be random. Some of the biotechnological problems associated with resulting position effects may be avoided by employing MAR like insulator or LCR sequences. However, from a practical and regulatory point of view, it is desirable to direct transgene integration reproducibly to defined sites within the genome. The tools of homologous recombination in embryonic stem cells (for review see Bradley et al. 1991) and the Cre recombination system (Odell et al. 1990; Dale et al. 1991) will aid us in our efforts to manipulate mammary expression systems. Homologous recombination in combination with the Cre/lox recombination system may also enhance our abilities to manipulate the mammary bioreactor concept. Upon introduction of a the 34-bp lox sequence either into the endogenous locus of a milk protein gene or into a locus permitting high-level regulated expression, it should be possible to use this site as an entry port for hybrid genes. Thus Cre-mediated integration of microinjected genes into the host genome should result in reproducible high-level production of foreign proteins. The "hit-and-run" homologous recombination technology should allow us to introduce hybrid genes into milk protein genetic domains. In the context of these loci the hybrid genes would be under control mechanisms identical to those of the endogenous milk protein genes. However, the realization of this concept can only be achieved with the development of embryonic stem cells from farm animals.

References

Andres AC, Schönenberger CA, Groner B, Hennighausen L, LeMeur M, Gerlinger P (1987) Ha-ras oncogene expression directed by a milk protein gene promoter: tissue specificity, hormonal regulation, and tumor induction in transgenic mice. Proc Natl Sci USA 84:1299-1303

Archibald AL, McClenaghan M, Hornsey V, Simons JP, Clark AJ (1990) High-level expression of biologically active human α1-antitrypsin in the milk of transgenic mice. Proc Natl Acad Sci 87:5178-5182

Bonifer C, Hecht A, Saueressig H, Winter DM, Sippel AE (1991) Dynamic Chromatin: The regulatory domain organization of eukaryotic gene loci. J Cell Biochem 47:99-108

Bradley A (1991) Modifying the mammalian genome by gene targeting. Current Opinion in Biotechnology 2:823-829

Brinster RL, Allen JM, Behringer RR, Gelinas RE, Palmiter RD (1988) Introns increase transcriptional efficiency in transgenic mice. Proc Natl Acad Sci USA 85:836-840

Burdon T, Sankaran L, Wall RJ, Spencer M, Hennighausen L (1991a) Expression of a whey acidic protein transgene during mammary development:

Evidence for different mechanisms of regulation during pregnancy and lactation. J Biol Chem 266:6909-6914

Burdon T, Wall RJ, Shamay A, Smith GH, Hennighausen L (1991b) Overexpression of an endogenous milk protein gene in transgenic mice is associated with impaired mammary development and a milchlos phenotype. Mech of Dev 36:67-74

Choi T, Huang M, Gorman C, Jaenisch R (1991) A generic intron increases gene expression in transgenic mice. Mol and Cell Biol11:3070-3074

Clark AJ, Bessos H, Bishop JO, Brown P, Harris S, Lathe R, McClenaghan M, Prowse C, Simons JP, Whitelaw CBA, Wilmut I (1989) Expression of human anti-hemophilic factor IX in the milk of transgenic sheep. Biotechnology 7:487-492

Dale EC, Ow DW (1991) Gene transfer with subsequent removal of the selection gene from the host genome. Proc Natl Acad Sci USA 88:10558-10562

Denman J, Hayes M, O'Day C, Edmunds T, Barlett C, Hirani S, Ebert KM, Gordon K, McPherson JM (1991) Transgenic expression of a variant of human tissue-type plasminogen activator in goat milk: purification and characterization of the recombinant enzyme. Bio/Technology 9:839-843

Ebert KM, Selgrath JP, DiTullio P, Denman J, Smith TE, Memon MA, Schindler JE, Monastersky GM, Vitale JA, Gordon K (1991) Transgenic production of a variant of human tissue-type plasminogen activator in goat milk: Generation of transgenic goats and analysis of expression. Biotechnology 9:835-838

Furth PA, Shamay A, Wall RJ, Hennighausen L (1992) Gene transfer into somatic tissues by jet injection, submitted

Gordon K, Lee E, Vitale JA, Smith AE, Westphal H, Hennighausen L (1987) Production of human tissue plasminogen activator in mouse milk. Biotechnology 5:1183-1187

Grosveld F, van Assendelft BG, Greaves DR, Kollias G (1987) Position-independent, high level expression of the human β-globin gene in transgenic mice. Cell 51:975-985

Hennighausen L (1990) The mammary gland as a bioreactor: Production of foreign proteins in milk. Protein Expression and Purification 1:3-8

Hennighausen LG, Sippel AE (1982a) The mouse whey acidic protein is a novel member of the family of "four-disulfide core" proteins. Nucleic Acids Res 10:2677- 2684

Hennighausen LG, Sippel AE (1982b) Characterization and cloning of the mRNAs specific for the lactating mouse mammary gland. Eur J Biochem 125:131-141

Hennighausen L, Westphal C, Sankaran L, Pittius CW (1988) Regulation of expression of milk protein genes. In: First and Haseltine (eds) Transgenic Technology in Medicine and Agriculture, Butterworth, 61-70

Hobbs AA, Richards DA, Kessler DJ, Rosen JM (1982) Complex hormonal regulation of rat casein gene expression. J Biol Chem 257:3598-3605

Krimpenfort P, Rademakers A, Eyestone W, van der Schans A, van den Broek S, Kooiman P, Kootwijk E, Platenburg G, Pieper F, Srijker R, de Boer H (1991) Generation of transgenic dairy cattle using "in vitro" embryo production. Biotechnology 9:844-847

McKnight RA, Shamay A, Sankaran L, Wall RJ, Hennighausen L (1992) Matrix attachment regions impart position independent regulation of a tissue specific gene in transgenic mice. Proc Natl Acad Sci USA

Odell JT, Caimi PG, Sauer B, Russell SH (1990) Mol Gen Genet 223: 369-378

Overbeek PA, Aguilar-Cordova E, Hanten G, Schaffner DL, Patel P, Lebovitz RM, Lieberman MW (1991) Coinjection strategy for visual identification of transgenic mice. Transgenic Res 1:31-37

Palmiter R, Sandren E, Avarbock M, Allen D, Brinster R (1991) Heterologous introns can enhance expression of transgenes in mice. Proc Natl Acad Sci 88:478-482

Palmiter RD, Brinster RL, Hammer RE, Trumbauer ME, Rosenfeld MG, Birnberg NC, Evans RM (1982) Dramatic growth of mice that develop from eggs microinjected with metallothionein-growth hormone fusion genes. Nature 300:611-615

Pittius CW, Sankaran S, Topper Y, Hennighausen L (1988) Comparison of the regulation of the whey acidic protein gene to a hybrid gene containing the whey acidic protein gene promoter in transgenic mice. Mol Endocrinol 2:1027-1032

Shamay A, Pursel VG, McKnight RA, Alexander L, Beattie C, Hennighausen L, Wall RJ (1991) Production of the mouse whey acidic protein in transgenic pigs during lactation. Journal of Animal Science 69:4552-5562

Shamay A, Pursel V, Wall R, Hennighausen L (1992a) Induction of lactogenesis in transgenic virgin pigs: evidence for gene and integration site-specific hormonal regulation. Molecular Endo

Shamay A, Pursel VG, Wilkinson E, Wall RJ, Hennighausen L (1992b) Expression of the mouse whey acidic protein gene in transgenic pigs is associated with agalactia and deregulated gene expression. Transgenic Research

Simons JP, McClenaghan M, Clark AJ (1987) Alteration of the quality of milk by expression of sheep β-lactoglobulin in transgenic mice. Nature 328:530-532

Velander WH (1992a) Production of biologically active human protein C in the milk of transgenic mice. Biochemical Engineering VII

Velander WH, Johnson JL, Page RL, Russell CG, Morcol T, Subramanian A, Wilkins TD, Canseco R, Williams BL, Gwazdauskas F, Knight JW, Pittius C, Young JM, Drohan WN (1992b) High level expression in the milk of transgenic swine using the cDNA encoding human protein C. Proc Natl Acad Sci USA

Wall RJ, Pursel VG, Shamay A, McKnight RA, Pittius CW, Hennighausen L (1991) High-level synthesis of a heterologous milk protein in the mammary gland of transgenic swine. Proc Natl Acad Sci USA 88:1696-1700

Wilmut I, Archibald AL, McClenaghan M, Simons JP, Whitelaw CBA, Clark AJ (1991) Production of pharmaceutical proteins in milk. Experientia 47:905-912

Wright G, Carver A, Cottom D, Reeves D, Scott A, Simons P, Wilmut I, Garner, Colman A (1991) High level expression of active human alpha-1-antitrypsin in the milk of transgenic sheep. Biotechnology 9:830-834

Yang NS, Burkholder J, Roberts B, Martinell B, McCabe D (1990) In vivo and in vitro gene transfer to mammalian somatic cells by particle bombardment. Proc Natl Acad Sci USA: 87:9568-9572

9 Targeted Inactivation of the Muscle Regulatory Genes Myf-5 and MyoD: Effect on Muscle and Skeletal Development

Michael A. Rudnicki, Thomas Braun, Hans-Henning Arnold, and Rudolf Jaenisch

9.1 Introduction

MyoD is a member of a family of myogenic transcription factors with similar properties [1] including myogenin [2–4], Myf-5 [5], and Myf-6, also called MRF4 or herculin [6–8]. Transfection of the myogenic HLH genes into a wide range of cultured cells can induce the skeletal muscle differentiation program and activate muscle-specific genes. No substantial difference between the myogenic HLH genes has been revealed by these assays. The myogenic transcription factor genes are expressed solely in skeletal muscle, and thus, their role appears to be in determining the identity of the skeletal myocyte lineage [9–12].

In vertebrates, skeletal muscle originates from a small pool of progenitor cells that arise in the early somite. These premyoblast stem cells become the dermamyotomal compartment of the maturing somite, from which myoblasts expand into the developing embryo. In mice, skeletal muscle development occurs in several phases. First to differentiate in the fetus at 8.5 days of gestation are the myotomal fiber precursors, which give rise to small spindle-like myotomal fibers displaying the earliest expression of muscle-specific genes. Starting around day 13 of gestation, primary multinucleated muscle fibers form in trunk and limbs and at day 16 secondary muscle fibers also begin to develop within the same basal lamina of the primary fibers. Throughout this developmental program, the myogenic HLH genes are activated consecutively [12], and this sequential activation suggests that they may have distinct functions in the developmental activation of the muscle differentiation program.

We have been interested in studying the role of the myogenic HLH transcription factors in muscle development. For example, are these genes functionally redundant, as has been suggested in a variety of in vitro assays? Alternatively, do they play distinct roles in progenitor commitment, myoblast proliferation, terminal differentiation, and in the maturation and regeneration of skeletal muscle? We have employed gene targeting in embryonic stem (ES) cells to begin a genetic dissection of the roles of the different myogenic factors in myogenesis. Mice lacking a functional Myf-5 or MyoD were derived and analyzed to detect any alteration in muscle development. Surprisingly, inactivation of either gene allowed apparently normal muscle development, supporting the notion of partial functional compensation between the different myogenic factors. Mutant mice lacking MyoD were viable and fertile, and exhibited no discernable abnormalities in skeletal muscle. Contrary to our expectation, however, homozygous Myf-5 mutant mice exhibited a severe skeletal defect, in which the distal part of the ribs failed to form. The lack of a defined rib-cage in these mice prevents the inflation of the lungs and leads to immediate postnatal mortality. In this review we briefly summarize our first analyses of these mutations. Details of the experimental results can be found in [13] and [14].

9.2 Results

9.2.1 Targeted Disruption of the Myf-5 and MyoD Gene in ES Cells

The genes were targeted using established procedures [15] in the J1 embryonic stem cells developed previously in this laboratory [16]. Both genes are comparatively small containing three exons—with exon 1 coding for the basic and HLH domains. The Myf-5 gene was disrupted by inserting a PGK-1 promoter–neo gene cassette into a unique ScaI restriction site located in exon 1, upstream of the bHLH domain [13] while the MyoD gene was inactivated by deleting the MyoD promoter and exon 1 [14]. ES cell clones carrying a disrupted Myf-5 or MyoD gene, respectively, were identified and injected into host blastocysts. The resulting chimeric mice transmitted the mutant alleles through the germline and mouse strains carrying either the disrupted Myf5 gene (designated as Myf-5^{m1} allele) or the disrupted MyoD gene (designated as MyoD^{m1} allele) were derived.

9.2.2 Lack of Myf-5 But Not of MyoD Results in Perinatal Lethality

Animals homozygous for the mutant alleles were generated by crossing heterozygous parents. When analyzed at birth, the expected number homozygous for either mutation were observed. Homozygous pups were of normal size and showed normal movements, suggesting no major disturbance of muscle function. While apparently healthy adults carrying two MyoD^{m1} alleles were readily observed, all mice homozygous for the Myf-5^{m1}allele died within minutes after birth. Affected homozygous Myf-5^{m1} pups failed to breathe and close examination of the lungs revealed the lack of ventilated areas. No other differences in comparison to their wild-type or heterozygous littermates were detected, suggesting respiratory failure as cause of death. Removal of the skin from the anterior thorax wall revealed a completely fused sternum with no recognizable connections to the ribs. The cranial rib stumps on both sides of the vertebral column ended in dilated enlarged structures which were likely to represent the remnants of the costovertebral joints. H&E staining of appropriate tissue sections revealed that homozygous Myf-5^{m1} animals contained striated muscles in the anterior and lateral thoracic wall and surrounding the rib stumps. However, the organization of individual muscles appeared disturbed, probably due to the lack of distal ribs. No abnormalities were detected in bones of the limbs, the head, the scapula, the clavicula, or the pelvis.

9.2.3 Mice Lacking Myf-5 or MyoD Do Not Exhibit Deficits in Skeletal Muscle

To assess possible structural defects in skeletal muscle of mutant mice, we examined tissue sections by light and electron microscopy. At low and high magnification, H&E stained muscle sections from mutant mice were indistinguishable from that of control mice. Similarly, staining of frozen sections with antibodies directed against fast and slow myosin heavy chain, actin, titin, nebulin and desmin revealed no differences between mutant and control mice. Furthermore, we examined the physiological status of skeletal muscle in mice lacking Myf-5 or MyoD by differentially staining sections of skeletal muscle for myosin adenosine triphosphatase (ATPase) activity. This procedure differentially stains type 1 (slow), type 2A (fast), type 2B (fast), and type 2C (fast) fibers [17]. The proportion of fast and slow fiber types were identical between wild-type and mutant mice in different muscles. These results were confirmed by northern analysis of RNA from mutant muscle using a panel of muscle-specific probes. Finally, transmission electron microscopy revealed no ultrastructural difference between mutant and control sarcomeres. In summary, mice lacking either Myf-5 or MyoD displayed a normal skeletal muscle system with normal muscle morphology. Our results indicate that apparently normal muscle development can occur in the absence of these myogenic factors, suggesting that the role of either factor can be functionally compensated by the action of a different myogenic factor.

9.2.4 Expression of Myogenic HLH Factors in Mutant Mice

To investigate whether expression of any other member of the myogenic HLH gene family was affected by either mutation, we compared the level of each myogenic HLH mRNA in wild-type, heterozygous, and homozygous mutant mice by Northern analysis. While the level of myogenin, Myf-6 or MyoD was not affected in Myf-5 homozygous mutant animals, the level of Myf-5 mRNA increased 3.5-fold in mice homozygous for the MyoD mutation as compared to wild-type controls. These results suggest that Myf-5 expression which is normally suppressed by MyoD is upregulated in mice lacking MyoD.

9.3 Conclusions

Table 1 compares the phenotype of mice lacking either a functional Myf-5 or MyoD protein. Muscle development was not obviously af-

Table 1. Phenotype of mice lacking functional Myf-5 protein
($Myf\text{-}5^{m1}/Myf\text{-}5^{m1}$) or MyoD protein ($MyoD^{m1}/MyoD^{m1}$)

	Phenotype of mice homozygous for	
	$Myf\text{-}5^{m1}$-mutation	$MyoD^{m1}$- mutation
Viability		
Prenatal	viable	viable
Postnatal	lethal	viable
Phenotype		
Muscle		
Markers	wt	wt
Function	wt	wt
Expression of myogenic factors		
Myf-5	–	++
Myogenin	+	+
Myf-6	+	+
MyoD	+	–
Skeletal system		
Rib cage	Defect	Normal

wt, phenotype indistinguishable from wild-type mice; +, normal expression; ++, increased expression; –, no or defective expression

fected by either mutation. Whereas mice lacking a functional MyoD gene were viable and fertile, animals homozygous for the Myf-5^{m1} mutation died soon after birth due to severe skeletal malformation resulting in a nonfunctional rib cage.

9.3.1 Myf-5 Mutation

The musculature of newborn homozygous Myf-5^{m1} mice displayed no overt abnormalities by a number of different criteria, such as histological appearance, fiber type composition, and expression of genes encoding various contractile and other muscle-specific marker proteins. In early somites, however, the first appearance of myotubes as evidenced by the appearance of muscle-specific markers seemed to be delayed by at least 2 days in homozygous Myf-5^{m1} animals indicating that Myf-5 may, in fact, be required for the early stages of myogenesis [13]. The absence of an apparent phenotype in muscle tissues of newborn mice carrying the Myf-5 mutation, therefore, suggests an extraordinary plasticity in the formation of the myogenic lineage with the myogenic factors expressed at later developmental stages substituting for the absence of Myf-5. This notion is consistent with the observation that the expression of myogenic HLH proteins other than Myf-5 (myogenin, Myf-6, and MyoD) was not affected in muscle of newborn heterozygous and homozygous Myf-5^{m1} mice. This result is also consistent with functional redundancy in the control of skeletal myogenesis in which the absence of one myogenic HLH protein may be compensated by another factor of the MyoD family.

The main phenotype caused by the Myf-5^{m1} mutation was a major defect in rib formation. The identity of the ribs and the shape of their proximal remnants was not affected in Myf-5^{m1} mutants, indicating that Myf-5 does not convey positional information. We consider two conceptually different mechanisms to explain the Myf-5 mutant phenotype: (1) rib development may be altered due to lack of expression of functional Myf-5 in sclerotomal precursors of the rib rudiments or, alternatively, (2) the mutation may act in the early myotomal cells, disturbing a crucial interaction between these cells and cells of the sclerotomal compartment (for detailed discussion, see [13]).

9.3.2 MyoD Mutation

Mice lacking a functional MyoD gene are viable and fertile, and exhibited, similarly to Myf-5 mutant animals, no morphological or physiological abnormalities in skeletal muscle. Northern analysis with a panel of probes revealed no difference in skeletal muscle-specific mRNA levels between wild-type and homozygous mutant MyoD^{ml} mice. However, the amount of Myf-5 mRNA increased 3.5-fold in homozygous mutant mice, suggesting that normally Myf-5 expression is inhibited by MyoD. These observations are in agreement with the notion that Myf-5, myogenin, Myf-6, and MyoD are part of a complex auto- and cross-regulatory network in which the activity of one member regulates its own expression and/or that of other myogenic HLH genes. The unimpaired muscle development in mice lacking MyoD suggests that other myogenic HLH factors can substitute for MyoD function in development. The induction in Myf-5 levels in mice lacking MyoD raises the possibility that Myf-5 may be substituting for MyoD activity in homozygous mutant MyoD^{ml} mice. Clearly, the phenotype of skeletal muscle of mice lacking both MyoD and Myf-5 genes will be highly informative as it directly addresses the question of mutual functional substitution of these two myogenic transcription factors in myogenesis.

The viability of mice lacking MyoD is reminiscent of observations made in mice bearing loss of function mutations in a wide variety of genes, including those encoding β2-microglobulin [18], c-src [19], pim-1 (P.W. Laird, personal communication), En-1 [20], and the NGF receptor [21]. These animals are viable and either have no obvious phenotype or exhibit a much less severe phenotype than might have been predicted considering the postulated roles and expression patterns of these genes. Similarly, the majority of mice containing loss of function mutations generated by retroviral integrations do not display overt phenotypes (reviewed in [22]). Thus, functional redundancy may represent a general principle in regulatory networks controlling complex developmental processes. However, it is important to emphasize that the lack of an obvious phenotype in mutant animals kept under laboratory conditions does not constitute a compelling argument against a unique and indispensable role of a gene in the normal physiology of an animal. For example, MyoD is the last of the four myogenic HLH transcription factors to be activated in development, and thus, may be essential for regulation of growth and/or regeneration of skeletal muscle after birth rather than in the regulation of de novo differentiation of skeletal myocytes. Clearly, mutant mice will have to be analyzed under a variety of physiological stress conditions for unambiguously assessing the in vivo function of MyoD.

Acknowledgements. This work was supported by grants from Deutsche Forschungsgemeinschaft, Deutsche Muskelschwundhilfe and the European Community to H.H.A. and by NIH grants R35 CA 44339-05 to R.J. T.B. was supported by a short-term travel grant by Boehringer Ingelheim Fond during his visit to Boston.

References

1. Davis RL, Weintraub H, Lassar A (1987) Expression of a single transfected cDNA converts fibroblasts to myoblasts. Cell 51:987–1000
2. Wright WE (1992) Muscle basic helix-loop helix proteins and the regulation of myogenesis. Curr Opin Gen Devel 2:243–248
3. Edmondson DG, Olson EN (1989) A gene with homology to the myc similarity region of MyoD1 is expressed during myogenesis and is sufficient to activate the muscle differentiation program. Genes Dev 3:628–640
4. Braun T, Bober E, Buschhausen DG, Kohtz S, Grzeschik KH, Arnold HH (1989a) Differential expression of myogenic determination genes in muscle cells: possible autoactivation by the Myf gene products. EMBO J 8:3617–3625
5. Braun T, Buschhausen DG, Bober E, Tannich E, Arnold HH (1989b) A novel human muscle factor related to but distinct from MyoD1 induces myogenic conversion in 10T1/2 fibroblasts. EMBO J 8:701–709
6. Rhodes SJ, Konieczny SF (1989) Identification of MRF4: a new member of the muscle regulatory factor gene family. Genes Dev 3:2050–2061
7. Miner JH, Wold B (1990) Herculin, a fourth member of the MyoD family of myogenic regulatory genes. Proc Natl Acad Sci USA 87:1089–1093
8. Braun T, Bober E, Winter B, Rosenthal N, Arnold HH (1990) Myf-6, a new member of the human gene family of myogenic determination factors: evidence for a gene cluster on chromosome 12. EMBO J 9:821–831
9. Emerson CP (1990) Myogenesis and myogenic control genes. Curr Opin Cell Biol 3:1065–1075
10. Olson EP (1990) MyoD family: a paradigm for development? Genes Dev 4:1454–1461
11. Weintraub H, Davis R, Tapscott S, Thayer M, Krause M, Benezra R, Blackwell TK, Turner D, Rupp R, Hollenberg S, Zhuang Y, Lassar A

(1991) The myoD Gene family: nodal point during specification of the muscle cell lineage. Science 251:761–766

12. Arnold HH, Braun T (1992) Myogenic control genes in vertebrates. In: Wassarman PM (ed) Advances in developmental biochemistry. JAI Press Inc. USA, (in press)

13. Braun T, Rudnicki M, Arnold H, Jaenisch R (1992) Targeted inactivation of the muscle regulatory gene Myf-5 results in abnormal rib development and perinatal death. Cell

14. Rudnicki MA, Braun T, Hinuma S, Jaenisch R (1992) Inactivation of MyoD in mice leads to upregulation of the myogenic HLH gene Myf-5 and results in apparently normal muscle development. Cell

15. Thomas KR, Capecchi MR (1987) Site-directed mutagenesis by gene targeting in mouse embryo-derived stem cells. Cell 51:503-512

16. Li, E, Bestor TH, Jaenisch R (1992) Targeted mutation of the methyltransferase gene results in embryonic lethality. Cell 69:915–926

17. Bancroft JD, Stevens A (1990) Theory and practice of histological techniques. Churchill Livingstone, Edinburgh

18. Zijlstra M, Bix M, Simister NE, Loring JM, Raulet DH, Jaenisch R (1990) β_2-microglobulin deficient mice lack CD-8+ cytolytic T cells. Nature 344:742–746

19. Soriano P, Montgomery C, Geske R, Bradley A (1991) Targeted disruption of the c-src proto-oncogene leads to osteopetrosis in mice. Cell 64:693–702

20. Joyner AL, Auerbach BA, Davis CA, Herrup K, Rossant J (1991) Subtle cerebellar phenotype in mice homozygous for a targeted deletion of the En-2 homeodomain. Science 251:1239–1243

21. Lee KF, Li E, Huber LJ, Landis SC, Sharpe AH, Chao MV, Jaenisch R (1992) Targeted mutation of the gene encoding the low affinity NGF receptor leads to deficits in the peripheral sensory nervous system. Cell 69:737–750

22. Rudnicki MA, Jaenisch R (1991) Insertional mutagenesis. Genome analysis, vol. 2. Gene expression and its control. Cold Spring Laboratory Press, Cold Spring Harbor

GPSR Compliance
The European Union's (EU) General Product Safety Regulation (GPSR) is a set
of rules that requires consumer products to be safe and our obligations to
ensure this.

If you have any concerns about our products, you can contact us on

ProductSafety@springernature.com

In case Publisher is established outside the EU, the EU authorized
representative is:

Springer Nature Customer Service Center GmbH
Europaplatz 3
69115 Heidelberg, Germany

www.ingramcontent.com/pod-product-compliance
Ingram Content Group UK Ltd.
Pitfield, Milton Keynes, MK11 3LW, UK
UKHW020231080726
473059UK00001B/24